I Really Didn't Mean To Get HIV

By
Livingston N. Lee, Jr.
and
Maurice M. Gray, Jr.

Write The Vision, Inc.

Express Press, Lima, Ohio

NOTE: Sale of this book without a front cover may be unauthorized. If this book was purchased without a cover, it may have been reported to the publisher as "unsold" or "destroyed," in which case neither the author nor the publisher may have received payment for the sale of this book.

Published by Write The Vision, Inc.
Box 12926
Wilmington, DE 19850-2926
302-778-2407
writevision@netscape.net
www.ourchurch.com/member/w/writethevision

Library of Congress Catalog Card Number: 2001090414

Lee, Livingston N., Jr and Gray, Maurice M., Jr.
   I Really Didn't Mean To Get HIV by Livingston N. Lee, Jr. and Maurice M. Gray, Jr.- 1st ed
ISBN: 0-9700514-2-5

Copyright 2001 by Write The Vision, Inc.

First printing November 2001 by Fairway Press

ALL RIGHTS RESERVED, including the right to reproduce this book or portions thereof in any form whatsoever. Any such reproduction requires permission from the author and/or publisher.

Printed in the USA

Dedication

This book, this labor of love, is dedicated to the following:

In loving memory, to my nephew Gerard "Tiny" Yarborough, December 27, 1962- August 10, 1991.

To my parents, Livingston, Sr. and Marthalene Lee

To my two sisters, Margaret and Olivia

To my wife Marie, whom God brought back to me at the appointed and anointed time. I LOVE YOU!

To the members of the Lee family, who preceded Margaret, Olivia and Livingston in serving the Lord so that we could find Him for ourselves at the appointed time.

To those who are living each God-given day with this disease of HIV and AIDS.

To those who have fought the fight against this disease and have gone home to be with the Lord

A heart-felt dedication to our church family, Bethel African Methodist Episcopal Church in Wilmington, DE, particularly the members of the AIDS Task Force (ATF) and the Beautiful Gate Outreach Center.

To everyone who has loaned us their time, talents, prayers and encouraged this project of love.

Special Thanks

To God — THANK YA!

To my brother, who sat through many hours of listening to me share and watching the emotional roller coaster that comes with reflecting over one's life. Bro. Maurice Gray, thank you.

To Sis. Regina Gray for donating her time and talent as our proofreader.

To our pastor, Silvester Scott Beaman, and his wife, Sis. Renee Beaman, for their unconditional support.

To everyone who encouraged this project with their prayers or kind words when we needed them the most.

Table Of Contents

Our Prayer Of Thanks	i
Forewords	iii
It Can't Happen To Me	1
How I Got HIV Without Meaning To	5
Recovery And Restoration	13
On The Day I Was Told	17
Family/Disclosure	21
Addictions	27
Bondages	35
Guilt And Responsibility	41
One Day At A Time	45
Having A Bad Day	51
Knowledge Is Power	59
HIV And Working	67
Medical Information	73
Women and HIV	79
One On-One With Me: When I Look In The Mirror, What Do I See?	87
Prayer Changes Things	91
From The Faith Community: Birth Of A Ministry	97
I Want To Help But What Can I Do?	105
Afterword: Writing The Vision	106

Our Prayer Of Thanks — Livingston and Marie Lee

Heavenly Father, most loving and gracious Father, this past year (2000) has truly been a year of your faithfulness. My wife and I would like to take this time-out to pray to You and say THANK YOU!

Father, when I had given in to being an AIDS victim and not a survivor, You said "Son, not so," and restored my weight from 139 pounds to a present weight of 185.5 pounds. Thank ya!

Father, on Jan 13, 2000 when the liver biopsy I was given went wrong and the death angel was close, You said "Back off," and raised me from that hospital bed. Thank ya!

Father, You brought my wife from California to Wilmington after 18 + years of separation and restored our marriage. Thank ya!

Father, you blessed Marie and me with the renewing of our vows in Your presence on July 22, 2000. Thank ya!

Father, when You transformed the three rooms I was living in into a home where godly love is ever present, we say Thank ya!

Father, when you sent the finances when things were messed up, we say Thank ya!

Father, You were there once again as the death angel attempted to rub me out for the second time and you said "He's mine and I've got work for him and his wife," we say Thank ya!

Father, this servant's prayer of thanking You is the evidence that prayer does change things. We say in closing, Thank ya!

In Jesus' Name we pray

Thank Ya for our undeserved favor

                                                                Amen

Foreword I: From The Author

I'm 55 years old. I have AIDS, Hepatitis C and I'm diabetic on top of all that. Because of one of the medications I took for the HIV virus, I've developed neuropathy, which gives me intense pain in my foot from time to time because of the damage to my nervous system. With all that, there's a lot of medication to take, and a lot of things I have to do in order to stay healthy. If you focus on your medical condition and nothing else, sooner or later you're gonna start feeling down. I'm a witness to that!

The title <u>I Really Didn't Mean To Get HIV</u> entered into my spirit one evening while ministering in Wilmington. I was participating in a seminar at the Northeast Community center on 28th and Pine, and in the middle of my testimony, I said, "You know, I really didn't mean to get HIV." When I got home that night, it dawned on me that this was something that God was asking me to do. I do believe in my spirit that He called me to go back over my life and reflect on some things and some moments, and some of the people I've met along the way.

Even though all I had was a title, it was apparent that this was enough to shake up my spirit and know that God was seed-planting something. That something manifested itself first in reflecting over my life and then to share with others the truth, that we are never alone in this earthly walk no matter what we're up against, including HIV and AIDS.

The more I thought about it, the more the title became a part of my inner thoughts and my spirit. Please keep in mind that in my spiritual walk with God I had and still have an obedience problem with listening and following what thus sayeth the Lord. Am I relating to anyone?

I told my pastor what God had laid on my heart, and that I had no clue how to write a book. He told me to talk to my fellow church member Maurice Gray, Jr., because Bro. Maurice was a writer. I finally did that, and this book is the result of our obedience.

With any disease, we need something in our lives to hold onto. When Brother Maurice and I weren't working on this project, there was a void in my life. I didn't realize it until it was gone how much

I needed this ministry. God has given me this as a therapy for me as well as to help other people. There are people out there who need this because they don't have this kind of opportunity to share what they're feeling. I believe that now I need this ministry because it brings me joy.

Even when I wasn't feeling well, I felt joy when we were working on this book. I remember a day last year when I was really feeling bad, but I was happy anyhow because it was a day when we were going to do a taping session for the book. This book has been a therapy for me, to sit down and tell how it's been in my life. Not trying to figure out why or what happened, but just to tell it and to know that others are out there who need to hear it.

Anyway, this is the finished product, our labor of love. I pray that you're blessed by it, because Bro. Maurice and I surely have been!

Livingston N. Lee, Jr.

Foreword II: From The Co-author

My first exposure to AIDS was in the early 1980's. A skinny, leather-clad 23-year-old comedian trying to make his way in show business, burst onto the scene, and among the jokes in his now legendary first televised comedy routine was one about AIDS. Eddie Murphy described AIDS as "that new disease." He referenced it as something homosexuals have, and joked that "you better keep your wife away from her gay friends. She could be hanging out with her gay friend, at the end of the day she give him a little kiss goodbye and come home with that AIDS on her lips." His other comment that stuck with me was that "if you get it, you keep that (stuff) forever, like luggage."

I remember that well, because not too long after that, my Uncle Ronald came home from California to die. He was my youngest uncle, always full of energy and life, but now, seemingly out of the blue, he was deathly ill and nobody could or would tell me what was wrong with him. What I knew was that Uncle Ronald had something incurable, like cancer only worse. It was something that the doctors really didn't know how to treat. There was no medication on the market and no treatment that could even try to cure this mysterious thing that he had. Nobody came out and said it in my presence, but after he died, I figured out that the same AIDS that Eddie Murphy was making jokes about was the mysterious disease that claimed the life of my uncle.

I say all that to say this: AIDS is everybody's problem. I don't believe that there is anyone more who can honestly say that AIDS has not touched their family or circle of friends in some way.

As funny as they were at that time, Eddie Murphy's comments reflected the ignorance that did and in some cases, still does accompany this disease (in case you haven't heard, you can't get AIDS by kissing someone who is infected!). That is not a knock on Eddie; in fact, I'm grateful to him for helping bring this disease to the public eye, particularly to the attention of his huge African-American audience. Far too many of us in this age of enlightenment and of medical accomplishment don't know the basic facts about this disease that is spreading so rapidly into all aspects of society. This is not "that thing that homosexuals get" any more. This is a real threat to everyone, like it or not, and we all need to be concerned and most definitely, informed.

I'm thankful that God chose me to work with Livingston Lee on this project, because it will reach in its own way as many folks as Eddie Murphy reached with his comedy routine. Where Eddie Murphy made us aware of AIDS, I pray that this book God laid on Livingston's heart and placed in my hands will make us all, infected and affected, willing to learn about HIV, AIDS and everything we all should know about it.

Maurice M. Gray, Jr.

"It Can't Happen To Me" — Why It Can

HIV/AIDS in this new millennium is still here with us, and it's still on the move. People are still dying, still suffering, still uneducated and still afraid. Even now, despite all the education and ways to protect ourselves from this disease, people of all ages are still taking unnecessary chances. They're still figuring "It can't happen to me." Well, I was one of those that figured it couldn't happen to me — **but it did.**

It's so important that all of us get on one accord about this medical epidemic. There's a spirit roaming among us that has come to destroy God's people, and HIV and AIDS is just another demonic vehicle designed to "take us out." However, we must stand firm against it. The Bible tells us in Hosea 4:6 that our people "are destroyed for lack of knowledge." We know that this disease is running rampant. Now we have to act on that knowledge before we are totally destroyed.

I asked a group of teenagers recently, "Have you ever done anything in your lives that you had not meant to do?" There was an overwhelming response to this question. Most of the kids were honest, and they owned up to their bad decisions such as leaving school before graduation, having sex too young and doing drugs. Though they didn't mean to receive the consequences, they still came. They put their futures at risk by giving up on their education or by possibly exposing themselves to HIV and AIDS.

We must realize that the enemy operates from our thoughts. Before doing anything questionable, we first think about it. That thought is a seed planted. We water those seeds by reflecting on that thought, which allows that thought to grow into a vision, and then into an action. Letting those seeds grow is an opening for trouble. The consequences of these planted and watered seeds are what make us think, "I didn't think it would happen to me."

There's a slogan that I've become familiar with that helps me even today. "Think, Think, Think." It only takes a few seconds to stop and think, and to allow the consequences of our actions to become a seed in our spirit. Before the seed has a chance to grow, we must think through the possibility that it can happen to me. The choices we make can affect our entire lives and the lives of other people as well.

On the day that I was infected with this disease, it wasn't a conscious choice. I chose to shoot heroin, but I didn't choose the consequence. I didn't say to myself "I'll infect myself with HIV today by sharing a needle." However, that was the consequence of the choice I made that day, because I was thinking, "It can't happen to me."

A Scenario.

A 23-year-old college student is told that he is HIV-positive. Before this diagnosis, he dreamed of serving the Lord, finishing college, working a good job and having a family. Now, presented with these facts, there is no logical choice at that time. Fear and despair are his only companions. Suicidal thoughts might enter into his mind. "I'm going to die, but I don't want to suffer. I don't want to suffer." What led this student to become infected? Bottom line: the belief that "It can't happen to me."

What causes us to be affected by this person who is infected with HIV or AIDS? The thought that "It happened to him." This student represents our brother or sister, our father or mother. He represents our friends. He represents our own fears, shame and brings home the fact that we are not immortal. Death is an experience that we will all encounter. Do we not have control over how we die and how we live? Making wise decisions can give us a quantity and quality of life.

Why is God important in this? Thinking that HIV/AIDS only happens to others is a trick of the enemy, Satan. The scripture says, "He comes but to kill, steal and destroy." The consequences of this deception and his movement extend around the world, and the evidence is seen in the increased numbers of reported cases of HIV and AIDS, and the increasing number of deaths from it. There is evidence of how we are all affected when we share in the loss of family members and friends. The growing sense of isolation, pain and desertion, along with the grief that must be addressed, is all a part of the lack of knowledge of this disease.

Persons *in*fected and *af*fected need other people who choose to become *effective* in sharing the truth about HIV/AIDS. We need someone who is concerned, understanding, considerate and open to share our experiences. God places people in our lives to help us through situations such as this. If we are willing to learn about this disease and to admit that this disease affects us, and if we are willing to stand firm against it, we may be the ones God chooses to use. God knows the whole story, from beginning to end.

We all make choices. We can choose to become wiser about the decisions that we make and we can choose not to put ourselves at risk. **Do not be deceived.** It **can** happen to **you.** It happened to me, **and I didn't mean to get HIV either.**

Decisions

What led up to me being HIV positive? Several things. As I touched on before, lack of education, lack of knowledge of words, identity crisis, (who am I?) not knowing whose I really was (other than my mom and dad's). Who did I belong to, what did I belong to, what was my destiny, where was my dreams, where was my hopes? What happened? Where did I fall through the cracks? I had a college degree; what went wrong? How in the world could a person such as Livingston Nathaniel Lee, Jr. become HIV-positive? Because of his behavior and one decision. Choices, choices that we make, decisions that we make, and who we make these decisions with.

For those who might be blaming somebody for giving this to them, or even might be blaming God for this, stop right there. Except for those folks who were genuinely minding their own business and got this thing because their significant other brought it home to them or through a blood transfusion, we had a hand in this. Remember, AIDS means **ACQUIRED** Immunodeficiency Syndrome. It just don't jump on us; we have to do something to get this thing, and those who are not yet infected can do something NOT to get it.

I got it because I chose drugs and alcohol as a way of life. Some may have gotten it through continuous unprotected sex. Some may have gotten it not because they were particularly promiscuous, but because they chose to have that one sexual experience and that person happened to be infected. These are choices we made, and we have to live with the consequences of those decisions. I'm not saying this to beat on anybody, just to be honest with you. Remember, this is a book of truth and honesty.

It's important that we be reminded that there are a lot of things in our lives that we really didn't mean to do, and that we have no control over the consequences that follow. Things like drug addiction and alcohol addiction and sex addiction and all the other things that alter our minds and lead us into making bad decisions can be turned around. We just don't have to go there. We don't have to open that door. From teenagers to seniors, this disease is no respecter of who you are if you put yourself in the realm of risk.

The devastation of this disease is like addiction; **it doesn't care.** Anybody can get this thing, no matter what race you are or how much money you have. Drug addiction is a huge factor. If you're hooked on drugs, rich and poor alike, it can lead to making a bad sexual decision, which is one of the ways of transmission. The desperation of the drug can alter some of the things that normally you're not about. I know I bumped somebody's head with that one! Don't take it as an insult because if you remember, in the introduction, you were warned not to read this if you're not ready for the truth!

Maybe somebody hasn't heard that HIV is still on the increase. It is, because of the decisions we make individually. When they count us collectively, that's when the truth comes out. Hopefully, you will make a choice that you will not be in the number infected by taking the necessary precautions. **We can stop this thing in its tracks. It starts with us.**

How I Got HIV Without Meaning To

I mentioned before that bad decisions are the main cause of HIV and AIDS infection in my opinion. For me, that was the case. Because of the choices I made, I got myself into something that my big sister couldn't get me out of, that my mother if she were still living couldn't get me out of and that I couldn't talk myself out of. It set me on what I call my journey of journeys, and I'm still walking it now.

I knew a little bit about HIV and AIDS, but not much. In my neighborhood, we knew it was out there, but it was just "that thing" that gay people can get somehow and therefore, it was nothing I needed to worry about. It didn't affect me, it had no bearing on my life at all, so I thought nothing about it until it did affect me.

It first affected me through my family. My sister Margaret told me that there was a problem, a situation in my youngest nephew's life. Gerard (we called him Tiny) was sick with something and it wasn't going to go away. This was my first introduction up close and personally knowing anything about HIV and AIDS.

Hearing this about Tiny was like an eye-opener for me. Seeing not just somebody I knew, but a member of my own family infected with this thing made me begin to think about my possibility of being exposed to "that thing." I remember a feeling of "This cannot be" first and foremost. Whatever this thing is that I'm hearing a little bit about, it can't be entering into *my* family. My family is special. My nephew was gay and living that lifestyle, but it still didn't enter into my realm of thinking that this was one of the ways you can get it. That's how little knowledge I had of the disease.

Although my addictive behavior, my IV drug use, had put me at risk, I was not aware that I **was** at risk. I know that this is year 2001, but I'm sure there are some folks out there that can relate to this even now. It's a dangerous thing, being at risk but not really knowing or thinking it through that you are putting yourself at risk.

So time went on and my acceptance of my nephew's medical situation became very real. My sister told me that the doctors had told her a very strange thing. The doctor said that Tiny only had approximately five years to live at the longest. Keep in mind I was still in active addiction and the day I heard this was probably one of those days when, if I hadn't got started yet, I was on my way to getting started doing what I thought I did best at the time, which was use heroin or drink or whatever it took to change the way that I felt.

When she said that he only had five years to live, I wondered how a doctor could say something like that to a mother about her child. Well, the doctors were right; he was only with us about four or five years after being told he was infected. At this point I didn't know the difference between HIV and AIDS; like a lot of folks do, I just lumped it all together. It was just this weird thing that had infiltrated our community.

I remember going on with my life, business as usual. I had a friend in my life, a young lady I was living with, and I remember during this time that for some reason, instead of me slowing down, my using picked up. I can't explain what my thoughts were because I didn't take out enough time to think things through as to why I was picking up my using. Was it the news about my nephew or was it just the progression of addiction?

I do remember this much. My friend and I, we had some difficulties at the time because I would continuously lie. That was a natural thing for me on any given day on every day; I would lie just to lie.

My girlfriend once gave me $240.00 cash to rent the room for her mother's birthday party. I don't know WHAT possessed her to do that. I saw that cash and all I could do was RUN for the bus and go to that neighborhood. I could be the man for a little while, until that money ran out. Then my "friends" were gone.

She called me later and angry wasn't enough to say how mad she was. She was like "If you were here, I'd KILL you. I'd get me a knife and — ." That's what addiction does to you. It makes you hurt the people you love most because it makes you totally selfish.

I remember her finally saying that she'd had enough and she put me out. Right around that time, my nephew was starting to get sick. My sister had decided that she didn't want her son to go into a nursing facility, so he moved in with her and I solved my problem by moving in his apartment, which was right down the hall from where my sister was living. That way, I had a place to stay and I could be available to help my sister with any situations.

This disease progressed real fast with Tiny. In a matter of two or three years, my nephew went from this healthy, very good-looking, young 28-year-old man to an individual that was basically skin and bones. And right around that time, my using began to increase. Tiny had a friend in his life that used also, so not only did I increase in my addiction, but I had a partner in crime, so to speak. I had company, I had someone to cosign on what I was doing, and tell me that it was okay and that it was fun

I remember watching my sister take care of my nephew as his health began to decline. She did have a business in her home, a daycare center, and I thank God for surrounding her home with His grace and His mercy. During that period, with the ignorance that all of us that I knew, and the lack of knowledge and the fear we had about this disease, my sister's business was still going on. Nobody pulled the plug on her business. Not one parent pulled their child out.

Somebody will relate to this, and perhaps somebody is going through this right now. Somehow my family got through it. As my nephew's disease progressed and he came to the point when he couldn't do anything for himself, my sister was getting strength from other sources. It was such a blessing (but I didn't know then that it **was** a blessing) to watch her on a daily basis take care of this gift from God, her child, her baby. I remember how much her love for her son seemed to increase, how she cared for her son, how he never missed a doctor's appointment. My sister was running on faith in God to help her on a daily basis to take care of her son.

This one thing sticks out to me. I still don't know why I did this, but I did. I had got started using pretty early that day, and I got on this corner where there was a telephone. I remember calling my nephew and I was whispering to him. These were my words.

"Listen, I don't want you to repeat this, but I want to tell you that nephew, I think, I'm not sure, but I think perhaps your uncle has gotten himself into a predicament similar to yours." Then I began to stress to him to please don't tell anybody, especially his mother. I didn't want to be an added burden with just my speculations at that time.

You know, in the place where I used my drugs on a daily basis, people were beginning to die. When I would ask what happened, the response was "Oh, they died from a heart attack" or natural causes. I said okay, that was good enough for me. But you know what? Something deep inside of me was saying that this disease we were periodically talking about, the one that Tiny had, now had infiltrated my life. I began to look at myself in the mirror one day and I don't know why, but for some reason the reflection was a reflection of sickness. My face had gotten awful thin and the jaw area was sunken in. That day as I looked at television, there was a commercial that came on about this disease called HIV and AIDS. For the first time I listened, just a little, not much. At that moment, for some unexplained reason, *I knew I had this disease.* Now keep in mind, at this time I was still very much in my active addiction. I was still back and forth with my friend, because she had forgiven me for the last situation. I'm back and forth from my sister's place to my girlfriend's. It was the strangest feeling inside me; I don't know whether it was fear, or a sense of "No, this can't be." I can't explain it, but I just knew something was wrong.

Life went on. I continued with the things I was doing, I helped my sister as much as possible and I still went out and got what I thought I needed on a daily basis. I got kicked out of my girlfriend's place again. This was an ongoing thing in my active addiction as I began to use more and more and more.

Remember now the statement that the doctor had made to my sister, and the time frame of my nephew's demise: five years. Within this five-year period, my life was being revealed to me, to some degree. I had periodically begun to think about things that I hadn't thought about at all: my health, things of that nature, but just briefly. I always managed to put it way, way on the back burner because I wasn't ready to deal with it.

My nephew's disease progressed so rapidly until I didn't even recognize him. I wonder how my sister made it through that period of the disease. For me, I had my drugs and my mind and mood-altering chemicals to take me out of the situation on a daily basis, not to have to really confront it.

I will never forget August 10, 1991. I got a phone call that an unemployment check had come to a friend's house. That's how unsteady I was; I really didn't have a permanent address to call my own so I had the check sent to my friend's house. I left immediately to get this check because I needed money to do my thing. This was the day that I will never, ever, ever forget, because this was the day my nephew went home to be with the Lord, **and I wasn't there.**

I had promised my sister that I would be there for her when it happened, because although I don't think I fully accepted it, this is something that was not gonna change. But the bottom line is, I wasn't there. I was out using. When I returned to the house, I looked at my sister and I remember not a look of disappointment, but a look of sisterly love for me even though I had broken a massive promise to her. She handled all of that with the help of other people around her.

My sister always does things that people will look upon and say she's crazy! At Tiny's funeral, she had all the family members stand in front of his casket and sing "It's So Hard To Say Goodbye To Yesterday." It wasn't a good day for me, and not just because Tiny was dead. I remember I didn't even have a suit to wear to my nephew's funeral. I borrowed a suit from a friend, and the suit was too big. I was in emotional pain and physical pain and I felt like I needed a shot of heroin to get me through the day. I was trying so hard to do this last tribute to my nephew without drugs in my system during the hours of the funeral, but man, was I in pain! I remember I was standing up there, thinking more about drugs than I was thinking about what was happening. I remember practically running to the drug man after the service was over with (isn't that awful?) and getting what I used to call "my medicine" to help me feel better. I don't remember where I got the money from that day, but I've learned that drug addicts can always manage to get a few dollars each day to get that drug.

Remember I said that this began my journey of journeys. After Tiny died, and how I was at the funeral, I began to think that perhaps I had a problem. I thought maybe I did have a problem with addiction, and perhaps I had a medical problem too. I thought maybe I could do something about it. Deep inside me, I wanted to do something about it, but I didn't know how to go about it because I was not familiar with the word called recovery. It just was not in the language of the people that I hung out with.

I remembered that from time to time, my dad, being a veteran, would go to the VA Hospital to deal with his drinking problem. Since I was a veteran too, I called our local VA and I got into what they would call a program. This was not my first exposure to it, but that's how the drug got me; to forget selectively certain things I didn't want to deal with. I'd been arrested for possession awhile back, before all this with my nephew. My sister had told me to go to a drug rehab and this would help me in court. I did that, but I was there for all the wrong reasons, and because of that, this was not in my remembrance.

In fact, while I was in the program that time, they gave me a pass to come out for a while. While I was out, I bought drugs and brought them back in with me. After they did what they had to do, to test me to see if I had used while I was away, I went in the bathroom and locked myself in a stall and I used, right there in the hospital, in the recovery program. Insanity! Can anybody relate? I'm sure they can.

So this was my second encounter with that thing called recovery. I remember my dad had gone in to deal with his alcoholism, to dry out from time to time, and I figured I could do that too. It was on the main floor of the hospital and I remember thinking it was funny that they would lock us in! How strange. I remember that I still didn't know why I was there. I thought they would give me some kind of pill that would make the addiction go away. But then we would have these morning meetings where we would just talk and share. Share what? Share my business? Oh no no no, I can't share my business. It's personal. I can't tell a bunch of strangers about who I am and what I've become. Because I was still kinda holding onto I was Joe College. I had a degree; I was a drug addict with class! The joke was truly on me.

I somehow managed to stay (I praise God for that) in the program long enough to go to the next level, which was to follow their suggestion to go to Perry Point Veteran's Administration Hospital and be tested for the AIDS virus. After being in that rehab program for two or three weeks, I was tested during the second or third week of October. I remembered counting the two weeks I had to wait, and one extra day because it was some holiday in the middle of October that delayed my results one day.

I remember getting the news from the head of the department and two counselors, one was my counselor and the other was there in case I fell apart. That was of one of THE most unheard of days in my life. But, it was a day I just didn't understand what they was telling me. Has anybody ever been there and done that? They told me that I was HIV-positive, but I still didn't have a clue what they were really telling me, other than I had this thing that we used to talk about in my community that was killing people.

This day is burnt in my remembrance; I will never forget it. I will never forget my reaction inside. My machismo may have shown outside, but I remember how I felt inside. And I still share that today with people; I had finally done something that was not gonna be reversed, by anything. I had this thing that was taking people out. Plus, now people were gonna think that I was gay! Aw, man! I didn't even know that you could get it from a needle. The joke was truly on me, because I had NO information. Would that have been a deterrent for me, to not use my heroin intravenously? I'll never know. But I do know this. There was a stigma that went along with HIV-positive in my community, and I had to come to some kind of terms with that, and I never did. It was just like a one day at a time process, without me acknowledging it. Just whatever's gonna be, is gonna be. I had done something that resulted in me not being in control, but I didn't want to give up the control I thought I had.

I went through the rest of the program. They kept me over a few extra days to get me stable. I remember that when I left the rehab that Friday, people in the program made me feel so good. I don't know where I got the strength from, but I told them, a bunch of strangers in this rehab I was in, what was going on. I remember that no one rejected me openly. Ain't that something? I'm sure there are people reading this who are saying, "Man, was he blessed!"

One incident stands out to me. During my stay in the rehab I had given a brother a bar of soap or something and the day that I was leaving, he couldn't be there, but he left me a letter. He said what a nice person I was and he wanted to say goodbye to me and how sorry he had to miss our round table discussion. I remember crying so hard that day. I remember being so encouraged and fired up, that I wasn't gonna use drugs any more and I was gonna do all this stuff. You know what? By four o'clock on that same day in the city of Baltimore, I used. I went back to what I knew best, and I stayed on the using journey for three and a half months, until I arrived back in the rehab on February 16, 1992. That was the last day I used drugs. I got back on track that day, and I have nearly ten years clean and sober now.

This is how I got HIV without meaning to. Does it sound anything like your story? It might. Does it sound nothing like your story? That might be the case too, and if so, I'm not surprised. However we all got this thing, it's in our lives now and we have to deal with it. Denial isn't the way. We have to face reality; we have to learn what we have to learn to take care of ourselves.

I'm remembering how some of the decisions we make even today have consequences we might not know about for awhile. With HIV, we can make a decision today and not know the consequences for months, or even years. Families are being stopped; bloodlines are being cut off because of this thing. Our grandchildren might be getting this.

When you know that we have the power — we have the power to do this. We can stop this thing. We can't count on anybody else to do it for us.

Recovery And Restoration

Getting it together after all my time being in active addiction wasn't easy. I mentioned how I decided to get clean, left the rehab and used that same day! Well, like I said, it took me another three months to try rehab again.

I remember coming back to the same rehab, seeing the same counselors and they didn't greet me with open arms! Oh man, what a letdown. That was okay though, because I had me an agenda. I had made up my mind that I was coming back to the rehab not to deal with my addiction, but to get paid. You see, I was a Vietnam era veteran, and I had heard that if you went through the program and got sent to the program at Coatesville, that you got paid all of this money. I was determined to get this money. This is when God began to slowly reveal Himself to me.

I didn't share with this community in Perryville (where I ended up instead of Coatsville!) about being HIV-positive because I was into "It's none of their business," but I was busting to tell somebody because it was overwhelming, this secret I had. And one day I was walking across the field to lunch with two other brothers and out of the blue I just told them. I said that I was HIV-positive, and both of these brothers were too! This was my introduction to God. What's the likelihood of me sharing that I was HIV-positive and not just one, but two other people I was walking with, the only two people, being HIV-positive too? God was holding me, and I didn't have a clue.

A friend sent me some music on a cassette tape, and one of the songs was "I've Been Redeemed," and I didn't even know what the word redeemed meant. I just knew that when I heard this song, it meant something to me. I didn't know how to inquire to what I was feeling inside. That's why nobody can ever tell me that there isn't a God. He really stepped up His love for me, during this, my second time around in the rehab. I finally let go of the money thing and I began to think that perhaps I didn't know what I was doing with my life after all.

The next day I was in a small group setting and this guy who was my counselor from before called me out. It was my turn to be on what we called the "Hot Seat" — this is when you talk and everybody else listens. This is something we had established for our small group. I was just talking and this counselor crossed his legs in my direction so that I could see his rear end and said to me "You were lying then, and you are lying now. YOU ARE A LIAR." I couldn't believe that this man was saying this to me. I called myself being honest — ha! He smoked me out. I wasn't serious about recovery; I was a liar who just hadn't had drugs in a few days. And I remember after the group I said "You know what? He called me a liar. I'm gonna make him a liar. I'm gonna get this recovery thing they're talking about because he called me a liar. He embarrassed me, he chumped me down, he made me feel like a punk in front of everybody, and I ain't having it! I'll show him!"

He sure tricked me, but it's the best trick that has ever happened in my life. Ain't that something? He called me a liar, and to make *him* the liar, I began to on a daily basis learn about the disease called addiction, I put down my hidden agenda about making a killing and stuff and my journey of journeys (even though it was slow motion), took off. I arrived in Wilmington, DE on 3/24/92, to the Salvation Army Rehabilitation Center. I shared with the intake worker about my medical status immediately, and he said it didn't make a difference.

On July 27, 1992 I was elevated to employee status at the SA as resident house manager. Remember, I was only clean and sober four months. I felt like I was the man!

On a daily basis, I would get up early in the morning, because I'd listened to a tape where the preacher said that this man named Jesus got up early before things started stirring around.

I had connected finally with the clinic at the Elsmere VA and I met this wonderful nurse and this wonderful doctor. As Pastor Beaman would say, my "edjumacation" with HIV and AIDS began, and I began to draw closer and closer to this living God.

I was invited to an afternoon service at a local church called Bethel AME by sister Joan Shaw. From then on, I began coming to the 8:00 service, and my journey with my church family began.

Over the years that I have been under the authority of God, there have been ups and downs. I've fallen sometimes and didn't get up right away. Sometimes I wallowed in self-pity. Sometimes I had disappointment with medicine not working, medical situations like diabetes and neuropathy, friends telling me that they were infected, etc. The stories, the testimonies go on and on in my life.

I didn't mean for any of this to happen, but had it not been for this disease entering my life because of my behavior, I don't even want to think where I would be now, or if I would still be anywhere alive. You see, what we sometimes meant to turn out one way, often can be turned around with God in the driver's seat.

On The Day I Was Told

I just came from a service and it gave me a little bit to work on. The sermon title was "Y'all Gonna Make Me Lose My Mind." As I was walking from Ezion-Mt. Carmel (where the service was) to Bethel today, I was thinking of how this relates to HIV and AIDS. We stand in agreement that we didn't mean to acquire this disease, but through our behaviors, we have it. The pastor really planted that thought in me (with that sermon) and I'm sorting through my thinking as to how a person going through can think they've lost their complete mind.

On the day a person is told they are HIV or AIDS; those of you who are with me in this thing, think back to that day when you received that news, that word. Were you about to lose your mind? On the day that I was told, even though I had a slight foreknowledge that there might be a problem, I wasn't pleased. Let me give you a description of what led up to that.

I had decided that when I came into the recovery process in a rehab, that I would be tested. On that morning when the counselor approached me and said it's time to go to the hospital to draw the blood, I remember vividly turning to the wall in the hallway of that rehab and just hitting my head against that wall. I was saying to my counselor that maybe I had changed my mind. I just didn't want to know definitely, even though my suspicions were very high. I'm sure someone is relating to this.

After my counselor reminded me that today was the day that I was going to be tested, and after banging my head against the wall like a crazy person, I finally conceded that okay, I'm going. I wasn't sure if I needed to know or wanted to know, but I went. I went on over, they drew the blood and that was it.

On the day I knew the word was back, I had passed my counselor in the hallway and he said "I'll talk to you later." But I knew what was getting ready to take place. In fact, I kind of knew what the answer was. I remembered sharing with my nephew on the phone that day in Baltimore a secret of my suspicions. When the true word came to me through my being tested, I thought I was going to lose my mind. Can you relate to this? I knew that this was one of the rare things in my life that I had acquired that I couldn't change. My momma and daddy had gone home to be with the Lord, and I had my older sister who could work miracles through her prayer power, but that wasn't going to change the words I was about to hear. This is not a put-down of the power of prayer — she knew to continue to pray for me through this storm and that it didn't have to be a death sentence.

I had thought I was gonna lose my mind waiting for the results to come in and already sort of knowing the answer. It's like knowing someone, a loved one, is going to pass away, but when you get that call that it has taken place, sometimes denial and non-acceptance of those words can cause chaotic dilemmas inside a person. That's what happened to me over that two weeks and one day period.

I was thinking all this as I sat in this room with these strangers and they shared this information with me. I absorbed it kind of instantly, but for some of us, it takes years to really accept it. Sometimes non-acceptance of certain things and situations in our lives really does give us an attitude of craziness. Some of us have chosen to continue on the road we're on, some of us have chosen to try to turn it around, some of us have chosen to be silent about it. There are so many different bondages with this disease, and I might not touch on all of them here. I'm hoping that at least I'll encourage you a little.

"Livingston Lee, the results have come in and they say you are HIV-positive."

Just like in a skit we do in the Aids Task Force, it got silent in that room. They allowed me to be the first one to speak after they said what they had to say. When they told me, the news went somewhere in my inner being, but I don't know where. I just took it in and didn't think about it too much. That's a very strange thing to think of. I didn't think I was like that. I didn't think I was living a secret life, but I was. I was telling people "I'm okay, I'm okay" when deep down inside I was screaming.

For the one who may be about to hear these words, I can't tell you how to prepare, or how you will react. I don't have that answer. I do know this. You sit and you listen, you hear what's being said and you go from there. What else can you do? It ain't gonna change. You can be retested, and get the same result. Someone has done that, I know they have, because they didn't want to believe the first result. "I ain't done nothing to get this thing." It only takes one time to turn your life completely around.

Losing your mind until you reach the point of acceptance can happen. With acceptance for me came peace of mind. I began to learn how to apply that to other areas of my life, such as accepting certain side effects of medication and accepting the fact that some people are afraid of HIV and AIDS.

There are solutions to every problem and situation. I encourage you, try not to lose your mind. Try to accept the situation at your pace. To those who will be getting that word, or have recently gotten it, I'm in my eighth year. It hasn't been a bed of roses, but it's been a blessing in my particular life. I won't tell anyone to take this road to be blessed by God, but through this, God has given me peace that surpasses all understanding.

Be encouraged. If you have decided to be tested and if you're in your two-week waiting period (or two weeks and a day maybe!), we do have commonalities. We're presented with circumstances that we can't buy our way out of. I think of Rock Hudson, the actor. He had all that money, but he couldn't buy his way out of this disease. Money allows you to be more comfortable in this thing, but it can't buy you out of it.

You didn't mean for this to happen. As soon as you can muster up the strength, move forward. Get some education on this thing. I pray that those of you who are about to be tested get a negative result. I advise that you practice abstinence for at least six months if you're unsure.

Don't lose your mind, absorb the information and get into acceptance as soon as possible so you can get the restoration of your peace of mind. Once you get that, then you can really get worked on medically and spiritually. If you're able to do so, share with others what you learn.

I touched on disclosure in another chapter, but part of that comes under this heading as well. When you're diagnosed with this disease, how do you tell your significant other? The devastation of telling your wife has to be one of the most difficult things a man can share, no matter what his age. I have been blessed in that area. My wife already knew my circumstance when she came back into our marriage.

Another thing that can make you lose your mind is the thought that you may have been infected with this disease even though you did nothing to get it. In the early days of this disease, lots of folks got it through blood transfusions before good screening and testing methods were available.

It may have been our fault. "If you'd never started taking drugs, if you'd never started drinking, this wouldn't have happened." Well, it did. I'm hoping that we can begin to get past the "if's" and get on to acceptance of what is. Ifs can really mess you up if you dwell in them.

I'll close with this passage from Matthew 21:12-13. Jesus came into the temple, saw that folks were selling stuff and corrupting the church and He just lost His mind. He started turning over the tables.

I say that to say this: sometimes it's okay to lose your mind, depending on how and why you do it. Sometimes it's difficult to receive certain information. Remember though, when Jesus lost His mind, He didn't stay there. Once the situation was resolved, He came back to Himself.

We have to realize that we are not in control. What we can control is the choices we make. Don't lose your mind. If you do lose it, come on back to reality and be restored to peace.

Family Ties

My family memories I guess are like anybody else's. I have good ones, bad ones and all in between. Some of it comes in bits and pieces, and some of it stands out.

I was born and raised in Baltimore City January 24, 1946 at 8:07 in the AM, the blessed son of Marthalene Lee and Livingston Lee, Sr.

I remember little things like sitting at the table being forced to eat oatmeal and I didn't really like it. My mom said "It's good for you, eat it!" And she was right — today I love oatmeal.

A big thing I remember is my grandfather dying in one of the projects that we lived in, and we had to go past his body to get to the kitchen and how scared me and my sisters were.

I try to remember sometimes what they call a normal family lifestyle with mom, dad and kids, but for the life of me I can't remember that happening. My father was always a part of our lives but he never lived with us. It was an off and on thing.

Being raised in Baltimore City was a good thing, due to the strictness of my mom. My mom was an alcoholic and my dad was an alcoholic, but somehow Mom managed to keep the three of us on track with positive thinking, positive things. As a child I remember her working for these white folks, Mr. and Mrs. Tompkins, cleaning their house. I used to go with her to do their windows every so often, especially around holiday time when special projects like that came up in the house. It gave me and my mom a chance to spend time. After we got off the bus, we had a long road to walk to get to their house. During those times, me and my mom really had a chance to just be alone, not have my sisters around, just talk to one another. She was a great talker. During those times she was teaching me how, as best she knew how to be a man, trying to teach me responsibility.

I was a very fearful child of school; bullies seemed to know they could push me around. In fact, I remember one time my sister had to walk me to school because I was afraid this one bully was going to attack me.

Growing up we lived in the projects. I just remember a lot of not haves, but my mom provided a lot of things for us. When school opened, we always had a new outfit, at least one.

I remember that my mom didn't go to church, but she would send us; me and my two sisters, one older and one younger, all five years apart. I remember being sent to Ames United Methodist church in Baltimore, for Sunday School. They used to make fun of me. I had this charcoal gray suit, and I think during those times I looked like a little midget preacher! I think God was trying to plant a seed in me even then. I wasn't listening though; I wanted to do some other things.

Later on, I remember my mom sending me and my two sisters to Macedonia Baptist Church, where my aunt (my dad's sister) was a member. I joined the usher board, tried to fit in but it wasn't working. We were baptized in that church, but eventually I strayed away.

How you're raised determines how you turn out. My mom and my dad when he was around did the best they could to raise us right. Mom was strict, but because I was determined to do my own thing and convinced that I wasn't gonna make it anyway, I strayed away from what Mom was teaching me.

I never felt confident or comfortable in school. The only reason I didn't drop out sooner then I did was because I knew what I'd get from my mom if I skipped! I managed to stay in school until 11th grade, and left then because my only son was created, Kevin Patrick Lee. I was 17, his mother was 16 and neither of us was ready to be parents. I know I was in over my head. I didn't know anything about being a dad. My dad had never been around to teach me- this is not blaming, this is just the facts.

I remember the friendship between my mom and me. It went so much deeper than the normal bonding between mother and son. I would share a lot of things with her, especially when I started to grow up and came out from up under her wing, a little bit. My early life, it was sort of protected by her; she didn't want me to do a lot of things most guys did. As a result of that, a lot of people thought I was gonna turn out to be gay because I had a lot of feminine ways about myself. Because of my upbringing with my mom,

I knew how to wash clothes and how to cook, I knew how to do a lot of things that women do, but I didn't know how to play basketball or baseball and those type of things. I felt like I had to find an outlet that would be acceptable to my peers so they'd get off me about maybe I was gonna be gay or something, and that was drinking. I started drinking early, with my cousin. She was a great teacher of drinking, and I thought it was fun.

There were just so many negative things in my life that I seemed to try almost anything to be accepted, which is why I kept drinking even when I didn't like the taste of it so much. And that, as much as anything else, led me down the path that put me where I am today. The only place I felt totally accepted was by my family, my mother and my sisters and that one cousin in particular. Once I had to step outside of that environment, I felt like I had to do something to belong, and I chose the same negative things I saw around me.

The decisions I made were in some ways influenced by my family life, but in others, were influenced by my peers. And even in the worst times I've had, my family has been my lifeline. My parents are both gone now, but my older sister Margaret has been there for me the same way Mom always was.

Disclosure

"Sharing With Others Along The Way"

I've had conversations with some brothers who are infected with the disease of HIV and AIDS. From these conversations, I'm beginning to learn from them different struggles that we have in dealing with this disease on a daily basis.

This last gathering I had with my brothers in Christ opened my eyes to the uniqueness of how each of us received the word that we were infected, and how each of us in this little small group of men began to share from our hearts what exactly was going on.

Our meeting was in the strangest place. These brothers and I gathered in the van God had blessed me with and we just began to share. I began to listen. As I listened to those brothers, I remembered a key thing the preacher said in a worship service I'd just come from. We have two ears, but one mouth, which means it's more important to listen than to talk. That really stuck with me through the gathering with these brothers. Even though I've become such a talker since I came to Christ Jesus, especially about the disease, I began to listen, not only to what the brothers were saying, but also to what they were NOT saying. Because of the Holy Spirit being in the midst of this gathering, I was able to listen instead of talk so much. As I began to truly listen to these brothers, I had such a sense of urgency in my feelings because for the first time I began to really realize that this small gathering of people was expressing themselves from inside rather than the outward demeanor that we usually display to folks we meet along the way, that macho thing, that toughness. I began to feel such a bond with these brothers. We became like family that day.

To paraphrase, nobody knows the troubles I see, nobody knows my feelings. Nobody knows what I went through immediately when I was told that I was HIV-positive, or again when I was told that I had AIDS. The day when I was told was a day in my life that I will never, ever forget. This gathering was another one of those days. Some of the feelings that I began to display in the gathering are feelings that perhaps I would have kept secret, maybe even taken to my grave. That's how I felt, that nobody else could possibly understand. These brothers do, and we needed to know that about each other.

To share one's inner feelings in reference to something this devastating is not easy, but it is necessary. We talked about a lot of things we had in common. You see, all of us have battled drug addiction at some point, and all of us made bad decisions. We stepped out and did things that perhaps we had no business doing. We were talking about specific incidences of things we chose to do in our active addiction, and then the subject came up of the day, minute and hour that we were addicted.

One brother held onto the fact that he knew the exact moment he was infected. I wondered then and I wonder now, is it that important to know *when* a person is infected? I've always thought that even though I didn't mean to receive this, it's not important to me when this took place. It was an interesting statement to investigate. Some folks can begin to focus on who did this to me, when did this happen, who's to blame? How consuming that can be! To be so focused on who committed the crime, to want to know who to blame. I'm sure that someone reading these words is perhaps going through this. It's my belief that, if we're to meet folks where they are in daily life, we have to know what's important. In cases like that, it's more important to listen than to speak. It didn't dawn on me that folks would be that consumed with how they received this disease, but it's real. Listening to those brothers really opened my eyes to this area of the disease.

I realized something important from that time of sharing. We're hurting, and maybe someone reading this is hurting too, so bad until they feel like they're the only one going through these things, these feelings. Your feelings are your feelings, and they're real because they're yours. Don't be afraid to reach out, to share if you've found brothers and/or sisters you can trust to listen and not judge.

The main thing that I came away from this gathering was the encouragement from a couple of them, and the discouragement that a few expressed. I shared with the brothers how hurt I was, how disappointed in myself I was, how easy it would have been to blame somebody else so I could have somebody to share this with. Such a deep hurt, such a deep disappointment. But, as I began to grow spiritually, I began to see that I had to learn how to be responsible for my own decisions.

A few years ago, two police officers came to a house in Wilmington looking for someone who they suspected of violating his parole. When they left that house, they saw smoke coming from the house next door. They went to investigate and found two guys in that house trying to dispose of a huge stash of marijuana! Apparently they saw the police coming, panicked and decided to burn the evidence! This is a clear (and funny!) example of how drugs take away your common sense and lead you into bad decisions.

Addiction

There's a definite correlation between drug addiction and HIV. Decisions are made under the auspices of drugs that can easily lead a person to becoming HIV-positive or to becoming AIDS-defined. A lot of us who are HIV-positive and AIDS-defined come from a history of addiction straight into this disease.

There are probably drug addicts who have been HIV-positive for years, but the drug in their system has been holding back any sick feelings, any warning signs their bodies might have been trying to send them. I know a few folks like that; once they got off the drug and got it out of their systems, their natural feelings came back again and then everything came down on them.

The ugliest thing you will ever see is a person, a drug addict with abscesses over their entire body. This is the destruction of God's temple; when you've shot up so much of a drug over time that you don't even have a vein anymore. I was in a house with a guy one time and he literally held his breath to make a vein pop up. I know of guys who even shot the drug into their penis because they didn't have any other veins left! If you're desperate enough to do that, you should start to wonder if maybe you have a problem, because you do! Remember, this is a book of truth and honesty.

On that note, I want to talk about a little bit about my addiction, and when it started in my opinion.

I remember being raised by my mom, as the middle child between two sisters. I was surrounded by three women all the time. There were early concerns that I might turn out gay because of the things I was taught in the home; how to wash clothes, how to cook; those were called woman things back then. Now these are all the things that I thank for God today, because I'm able to take care of myself by knowing how to sew cook, clean.

How did that label of people thinking I might turn out gay have an effect on my development? Was I becoming a product of the way someone else saw things? My mom taught me certain things, and even in active addiction there were certain boundaries I didn't dare cross. But there were also boundaries she told me not to cross that I chose to cross anyway. I guess that was rebellion; getting away from the apron strings of my mom, the domination of my older sister and the quietness of my younger sister. When things began to come in my path that I was curious about but I usually did not dare do because my mom had said "don't dare do that," there came a point where I chose to take the courage to rebel against what Mom had said.

I was thirteen or fourteen when I started drinking. I had a cousin that was a little older than I was but for whatever reason we became close. She participated in drinking, and she introduced me to drinking too. At that time we was drinking the common everyday wine: Thunderbird, Arriba, Gypsy Rose, those type of things. They had a powerful effect on me because I hadn't been exposed to that before.

We lived in East Baltimore and I had to walk all the way across the bridge to get to West Baltimore, but I did it every Friday after school just to hang out with my cousin. She would take me to the different places she would go and there would be drinking and all kinds of things I wasn't aware of or I had no knowledge of. If what they were smoking was reefer, I didn't know at that time. My knowledge of drugs and alcohol was very limited. My mom was a drinker and my dad was a drinker; it was ironic that I **didn't** have knowledge of drinking sooner than I did. My cousin began to teach me. As I read in the 27th Psalm verse 11 "teach me thy way," she began to teach me *her* way. I remember one time being so drunk that when they got me home, they stood me up in front of the door and rang the bell, and when they heard my mom coming they ran. When Mom opened the door, I fell on my face, literally fell on my face into the house. I felt real bad about my Mom being exposed to that part of me, but it didn't stop me. That was the beginning of me actively using something to change the way that I felt.

One of the counselors in a rehab I went to, Perry Point VA Medical Center, really got to the heart of the matter. He asked us as a group "Why did you drink and drug?" We had all kind of answers, but after we gave them, he began to open up and tell us why we drank: *because it changed the way we felt.* It really didn't make no sense until a few years ago when as a counselor at the Salvation Army I began to understand the point he was trying to get across. Obviously somewhere along the line, I wasn't comfortable with Livingston Lee. When my cousin came along, there was nothing for me to fight back that temptation with. This is no knock on my parents, but I didn't have any dreams. I didn't have dreams I could hold on to, to fight against going that route.

Maybe it sounds confusing, but I didn't have anything at that point. I wasn't deeply into school; I only went because I knew the punishment I'd get for not going. That was it though; I just went. Nobody around me ever said anything like "You are talented, you can be a doctor, you can be an attorney, you can, you can, you can." There was a lot of despair around me, a lot of hopelessness, and I don't think it was an intentional thing. My mom did instill positive things in me as best she knew how, but I was around a lot of negative things. The biggest excitement we had was to leave our home in the projects and go to the 500 block of Baker Street. While they drank, we sat on the steps or played or whatever until night fell and the fun really began. We really didn't need any TV because all the shows were on the streets of the neighborhood! There were people across the street fighting, ambulances, police sirens, all kinds of things happening. These are the sounds of the ghetto I lived in.

Drinking changed the way that I felt and it was fun. As the drinking escalated I began to act out. I wasn't violent or anything when I drank; the liquor just made me come out my shell. For example, I liked to dance, but if I was sober, I wouldn't dance. I liked to talk, but if I was sober, I wouldn't talk. I was very quiet and laid back, but the drinking made me this other person that people seemed to really like. They'd say "Oh, he is so *crazy!*" and this type of thing. I began to believe that I needed the alcohol to be a better person, and that put me on the path to my alcoholism.

Experiencing my first blackout should have been a sign to me, but it wasn't. Any time you have to ask your friends the next day what you did last night, you should be wondering if there's a problem, but I didn't.

I got married at seventeen because the young lady I was seeing at the time and I made a baby. By the time I was nineteen, I wanted out and I joined the Army. I went to Fort Jackson in Columbia, South Carolina and from there, I was sent to Vietnam. That's where the drinking really began to escalate. Of all the jobs for me to do besides my regular Army duty, I was the bartender! I worked in the club downstairs from the hotel where we lived in Vietnam. IW Harper and Seven became my best friend.

At some point in Vietnam, I was exposed to marijuana. It was a daily thing, just something to do. This is how the addictions escalated. I didn't see anything wrong with it. I figured it was the norm of military life and that I could handle it. After all, I was in the military and I was working every day and I was functioning, so in my mind, there was no problem with drinking and getting high.

I remember one time in Vietnam, one of my roommates (there were four of us to a room) said the VC (Viet Cong) were coming or something and I knew I was too wacked out to deal with something like that. Instead of cleaning my weapon, I took a pencil and covered over the rust! I didn't know whether the rifle was gonna blow up on me or not, and I wasn't really concerned. There were other "little" incidents like that which I never attributed to drinking and smoking marijuana until later. But, my time was so consumed with the drinking and the smoking until I didn't have time to do the things I needed to do, or learn the things I needed to learn. That was dangerous. I mean, what if the VC **had** come and my rifle didn't work? I didn't think like that; I just wanted to feel different.

Time passed and I made it home. The drinking got worse; like with all of us, they had sent a letter home from Vietnam to my wife letting her know that because of things I'd seen there, things I'd done, I might be different.

I was still trying to make this marriage work. My son was a beautiful boy, about one or two years old. I wanted so bad to be a dad and a husband, but the truth of the matter was that I didn't know how. I had learned so much about drinking and drugging that I couldn't fit anything into my mind about how to be a husband and a father. I tried to make the two intertwine, but it didn't work. One had to give, and I chose the wrong one.

I hung in there for a little while and then I reunited with a guy from Long Island. We had worked in a kitchen together in Vietnam, and while we were there, he said that if I ever needed him, to look him up. When things got really bad in Baltimore, I called him and looked him up. He invited me to come stay with him, and that was all I needed to hear. I packed my little bit of stuff and left. I arrived in Long Island, New York on a Friday night looking like a country boy! I had a hat on that was SO country, and my friend let me know it!

I thought moving to New York would solve my problems, but that wasn't the case. I found out that everywhere I went, I took Livingston with me. Until I started to address problems that I didn't even recognize as problems, nothing would change. Before I knew it, my stay in Long Island was just as bad as Baltimore because I didn't stop drinking and I didn't stop drugging. In fact, things were worse for me in New York because I didn't have any family around who even understood me a little bit. The drinking and the drugging continued, and after being there almost a year without that strong family support, I bottomed out.

It started off okay. I got there on a Friday and got a job on Monday making epoxy for the streets. I ended up working for the Post Office as a mail carrier, which was a terrific career-oriented job. However, my addiction prevented me from taking advantage of it. I'll give you an example. I had been drinking and I had decided that I wouldn't deliver the mail on the day it was supposed to be delivered. I took it home with me and I delivered the mail on Labor Day instead. Do you hear what I'm saying? *I delivered the mail on a holiday.* Of course people began to report, because their checks were supposed to be there and they weren't. Needless to say, I got fired.

I moved on to the mailroom at Chase Manhattan Bank, but that wasn't any better. For instance, working on the job, on the third day, there was a small demonstration of a play out on the mall in the downtown area, to get people to see what was happening and get them to come to the play. I remember stopping to watch, and I stayed out there so long that when I got back, they had fired me. This was on and on and on, and I didn't make the connection. I didn't stop and think that drinking and drugging was causing problems with me holding a job. All around me, my buddies around me managed to keep their jobs. What made Livingston so different? My best friend has worked the same job for twenty years and we drank together! His brother never had a problem holding a job, and he's still drinking! But I was the one who couldn't keep a job and couldn't figure out why.

Something broke down inside me about this whole deal. Working, drinking and drugging; somehow I knew I just couldn't do them together and be any kind of successful. I know in one year I went through twenty plus jobs. I would just work a week, get a check, quit. I'd quit over dumb stuff. These are things that I've gone through on the job now and I'd never quit because of them, but back then, I would quit

After that year, it was time to go back to Baltimore. My friend's mom, Miss Hazel, she was a beautiful woman. She adored me; she took me as one of her sons. She tried to help me, but I just wasn't ready to hear it yet. Being around her made me miss my family back home, so I decided to go back to Baltimore and try to live there again.

I got married again, this time to Marie. We're still married to this day, but it wasn't easy. The same things that killed my first marriage nearly killed this one too. Marie and I both drank, both smoked reefer and that was no good. Her brother sold it (God rest his soul), so we always had a supply on hand.

Marie had three sons and I had my one. I couldn't even deal with my one son and now I had three stepsons too, a mini Brady Bunch so to speak. I did the best I could, and then at age of thirty-two, I said I had enough of that and went back in the Army.

Notice the repeat performances in my life. When things got rough, *I ran*. Whether it was to the Army, to the bottle, to the reefer; I always ran to something rather than just deal with what was going on. Now I know that the ultimate price for my running was becoming HIV-positive. It was there, waiting for me to make that one decision to use on that particular day at that particular time so that I wouldn't have to deal with certain things. I ran to the drug one time too many, and that one time was the time when the needle was contaminated and I got infected.

I'm glad to be clean and sober for this amount of time (nine years now); it's a blessing from God. To be perfectly honest, I really enjoyed drinking, I enjoyed drugging, but I didn't enjoy the results. The headaches and all that stuff from the drinking, the soreness in the body from the heroin and the mind games that the coke played with me; to be controlled by something from outside of myself was not enjoyable at all. Some people say I'm being controlled by HIV now, but no I'm not. HIV is a controllable disease.

I was addicted to drugs and alcohol or anything that changed the way that I felt. I had to deal with that double whammy first so that I could go on living. First I decided that I wanted to live, and then I got greedy; I wanted to live a good, quality life. God saw fit to clean me up, to help me get free of addiction and to want to live and live well and to serve Him.

Now that I'm clean and sober, I can see things about being addicted that I want to pass on. For example, there is a certain trust factor that you develop as an addict that easily translates to having faith in God. We will give our money to a total stranger on a street corner because we have faith that they will deliver the drugs we asked for, yet we can't trust God with our lives the same way we trusted the dealer with our money. Hmm.

Another thing I know now is this. A lot of the liquor bottle labels have demonic symbols on them. We're basically being forewarned that we're about to take evil spirits into our bodies, but when I was out there drinking, I didn't have the knowledge to know what we were getting into. Hosea 4:6 again; "My people are destroyed for lack of knowledge."

If anybody reading this book has not opened the door to addiction: crack, heroin, alcohol, whatever, remember: *you don't have to*. It can take you on a journey that you won't want to travel. Drugs will have you standing at a family member's funeral and craving the drug more than you're grieving the passing of your loved one. It can have you crawling on your hands and knees to find something to get high off of, and stealing from a friend who has told you that you can have anything in their house if you just ask. It can turn you into a person who lies until you don't even know what the truth is any more. It can inflict on you medical situations that you cannot turn around through medication unless God Almighty Himself in His sovereignty decides to remove it. It can have you disrespecting not only yourself, but also the very ones you profess to love. It can have you make statements such as "Leave me alone; I'm only hurting myself."

Anybody ever said that before? Well, we're *not* just hurting ourselves. We're hurting our significant others, we're hurting our families and we're hurting society as a whole. Drugs, alcohol, they're not the answer. God is the answer; getting high or drunk only causes more questions.

For those who are addicted to drugs (and this is not a promo for this aspect, just a warning of how desperate we have become), I never thought I would hear in the USA something called a needle exchange program. We have this in some of our cities. Baltimore, the city I was born and raised in, has one. I went and observed how it works. I'm not promoting this; I'm just talking about this now because I want the reader to know that if your city doesn't have a needle exchange program, we can come up with our own needle exchange program within ourselves. If during the moments of your sanity before the need comes on you, you can prepare, do it. I'm not promoting drugs. I just want you to take precautions so that you won't be infected and you won't infect anybody else. The bottom line is that we need to go to any lengths as individuals to stop this disease. We're in the year 2001 and the disease is still growing. HIV ain't went nowhere, family; it's growing.

Bondages

Deep inside of me, I knew for a long time I was HIV-positive, but I set it aside. I was trapped in fear, that if I got tested I might find out for sure that I was, and I was scared to face that. I guess it takes being set free to realize that you are in bondage, because I didn't realize how secretive I was until much later.

When I did finally get tested and learned my status, I wouldn't talk about being HIV-positive unless I was pressed about it, like at doctor appointments. Other than that, I just didn't talk about it.

It's a universal thing with those of us that are HIV-positive. There is that bondage of fear attached to this disease, and it isn't until we're set free that we realize that we were even *in* bondage. I didn't know *I* was. Even in my drug and alcohol addiction I didn't know I was in bondage because for me, that was normal.

There are different bondages we experience by knowing we are HIV-positive. We go through a whole range of emotions and situations and such that are a part of this disease, and there's nothing wrong with that. You're not supposed to take this lying down. You have the right to be upset at finding out that you have something that will change your life forever. But you can't stay trapped in your sadness.

CHANGE: I knew I had to change how I was living if I was gonna get through this thing, but I didn't want to. Being an addict wasn't great, but it was what I was used to being. One of the big fears I had was this: if I change, who am I going to be?

My faith in God became quite important to me as I fought that battle, and Hebrews 11:1 became a verse I leaned on. *"Now faith is the substance of things hoped for; the evidence of things not seen."* I couldn't see it right then, but I began to believe just a little bit that the change would be better than what I had become: which was an addict.

My faith became sufficient, because despite all the aspects of this disease, all the feelings, all the tears, all the regretting, all the things that most of us experience, I finally knew the truth. I had to choose something, I had to change, and I was afraid. I was forty-seven years old at the time, and I was set in certain ways that I thought I couldn't change.

I use a slogan when I'm out teaching. "Liar, liar pants on fire!" My pants were **blazing**. I **could** change these things I was holding onto, but I just didn't want to. Fear was a big factor. Then I was introduced to the 27th Psalm, verse one. *"The Lord is my light and my salvation; whom shall I fear? the Lord is the strength of my life; of whom shall I be afraid?"* It became a personal thing then.

Sometimes you just have to step out on faith. Even though we can't get any guarantees like I wanted to submit to change, it was an absolute necessity for me to become a better person. What I had become- an addict- was not what God had designed me to be.

FEAR: There is a lot of fear connected to this disease. When we find out we have it, we're afraid we're gonna die. We're afraid people will treat us differently. The fear of how people will react to us when they find out is a big one. To share this kind of news with somebody is difficult to think about. It's not so much how many people you tell, but what kind of people you tell that makes the difference.

The day that God allowed me (though Pastor Beaman) to stand up in the pulpit of Bethel AME Church in Wilmington, DE to bring a word (from the book of James on how "the fervent prayer of the righteous availeth much") was a revelation. One of the thoughts I was having as I was bringing that word (and in the process, revealing in public that I was HIV-positive) was of one person: Sister Annie.

I sat with this woman in the eight o'clock service for over three years. She was truly my pew buddy on Sunday mornings because of her spirit. Our only interaction was church, but right then I was concerned what she would think of me. I wondered what she was thinking now that she knew I was HIV-positive. We had hugged often, and now I wondered if she'd jump up from her seat and go get a doctor's appointment that day because some of my tears had touched her at times, and she might be afraid that I had infected her. I didn't know what knowledge she had of the disease of HIV and I was very scared for her and scared for myself because I might be thoroughly embarrassed.

While I spoke, I searched for her in the congregation to make eye contact. I wanted to see what kind of a look she had on her face while I was sharing; if she had a look of fear or shock or if she was okay with what she was hearing. That was more for me than for her; I was very selfish in that. I wondered if God would allow me to read her face and know how she was feeling. He did, and I could see by the look on her face that Sister Annie was still my pew buddy.

Wondering how others perceive us before knowing and then how they perceive us after finding out that we're HIV-positive can put you in bondage to fear. You start to wonder what kind of struggles people have when they find out that somebody they know and have had a lot of contact with has this thing. Do they go "Oh my God, am I infected?" In talking to many people who are infected with HIV and AIDS, I'm finding just how many of us **still** refuse to tell anybody our status out of fear.

Another part of the fear bondage is the fear that you've infected someone else with this disease. My fear was for the woman in my life at that time. Remember, when I was first told, my first thought was "I've done something I can't reverse. My sister can't get me out of it, nobody can get me out of it." My second thought was did I infect the young lady in my life with this thing too? My sexual appetite was not all that great during the latter stages of my drug addiction, but we were together. I do remember her saying to me one time that we wouldn't do anything without me putting on a condom. At that time, neither one of us knew or suspected if I was or I wasn't infected. Knowing this person as I do, I doubt very seriously she had any education about HIV and AIDS. This tells me that God was in the midst of it all. To this date, there is no evidence that she's infected. Thank God.

PHYSICAL INTIMACY: There can be bondage in thinking that your marriage is over in a physical sense because of this disease. However, with this disease, one can still have a healthy sexual experience with their wife or husband. I spoke with my pastor about this, and he inserted the word intimacy into my spirit. Intimacy doesn't automatically have to mean the physical act. There are so many other ways we can show affection to each other. Just think on this. Say you have someone in your life who you love very dearly, who knows your medical situation and has chosen to stay with you anyhow. Think of how lovely it would be if he or she's employed, when they come home from work and after dinner, you prepare a nice warm tub of water. Spread some rose petals around, light a couple candles, maybe put some music on and just enjoy each other through touching and caressing.

Coming from the background of an addictions counselor, I've heard so many people say they're addicted to sex. Sexual addiction is a bondage. If you know you have that problem, then you need to take whatever necessary steps to resolve it. And while you're in the recovery process, *take precautions*. I don't advocate sex before marriage, but I do face up to the reality that people have sex before marriage. People who are infected and not infected do this; that's the reality of where we are in this world. The message is, we need to take charge and stop this thing. We can do it. We can stop HIV in its tracks. Remember, AIDS means **ACQUIRED** Immunodeficiency Syndrome. We have to do something to get this thing, and we can do something NOT to get it, namely we can practice self-control and abstain or we can use latex condoms to try and protect ourselves. We can stop this thing in its tracks. It starts with us. Hopefully, you will make a choice that you will not be in the number infected by taking the necessary precautions not to.

I say this because I want the enemy to know that we will not be defeated. There are ways to enhance life and not destroy it, and we don't have to be overcome and succumb to the flesh and take risks. All of us who are infected know that it only took one time for us to be exposed and get infected.

Be encouraged that HIV and AIDS, and I will always say this, we really didn't mean to get this, but we did as a result of our decisions. Please don't let it consume you. Don't let it be your demise. I have broken the bondage of fear by choosing to ask God to forgive me if I have hurt anyone along the way. I invite you to that same table; there's plenty of room to ask forgiveness from God. I also ask God to be with any person or persons I may have infected, to help them regardless of their choices. They might be still out there, they might be in denial after receiving their test results, but I ask Him to help them anyway.

Prayer To Help Us Go On: God, thank You for your special anointing. Thank You for loving us, for working with us and guiding us. Continue to bless us and our families, and all the endeavors you have chosen for us to do. In Jesus name, Amen.

Guilt And Responsibility

I paid $2.00 for my HIV status.

While I'm not sure the exact day and time it happened, I just know in my spirit that I became infected with this disease at the house where I did most of my using in Baltimore. Those of us who were regulars at that house had noticed for awhile that there was a high number of regulars who died and nobody thought it was strange. Looking back, I know why. All those heart attacks and "natural causes" that those people died from were brought on by HIV/AIDS.

The $2.00 I'm talking about is what it cost to use the house works. You could bring your own tools or if you didn't have any, you could rent the house syringes for $2.00. I paid the $2.00 most of the time.

Have you ever had a thought of perhaps how many people you may have infected before you found out? Talk about a heavy burden of blame. You can think things like "how many am I charged with? How many did I give this disease to before I knew what was going on? How many times did I re-infect myself with different strains of this disease? How many years have I taken off my life by not getting tested sooner?" If we choose to let it, HIV/AIDS can really open the door to devastating fears. That's an Arsenio Hall moment: it really makes me go "Hmmm."

For those who are in the process of retracing to find out if they might have infected someone and then wondering how to share with those folks, the question "What do we do?" is real. It can be a bondage if we let it. Now you know what your status is, you start wondering if maybe you and this person might have shared a toothbrush or did my blood get on her somehow if I had a cut? I know someone out there is going through this.

Retracing was a blessing for me. As I went back over my life before the time when I knew I was HIV-positive and thought about the possibility that I might have hurt somebody by giving them the disease, the possibilities were limited. However, there were two possibilities.

One was the woman I was seeing at the time I learned I was infected. I began to sort through "Did I infect her?" Thank God she got tested, and to this day, she has not showed any infection.

The second was because of my active addiction. For those of us who were into injecting drugs, how many times have we shared needles before we knew? For some of us, how many times have we shared a needle after we found out because everyone there was so anxious to get the drug in them? Being a former intravenous drug user, I can speak on this, and I think of one person in particular.

After I was told, I relapsed into active addiction. For three and a half months, I chose to go back to the world I knew, using alcohol and drugs. I went back to the area I knew, the house I always used to frequent. And, I went back in that room.

Lord help me, this person and I shared a needle. I did clean it, but did I clean it enough? This person was so anxious to get the drug in them. I remember it was just the two of us in the room. They were saying "Hurry up, hurry up!" Did I cleanse it well enough that they didn't get the disease? I don't know. I have had no contact with this person to this day, and it wasn't until today that I thought about it.

I can't remember if I had my own set of works that day or if I paid $2.00 once again to use the house works. I do know this. For a few moments, God forgive me, I did want to hurt somebody because I had this disease and I had zeroed in that I had got infected using house tools in this particular house. I didn't set out to intentionally use tools and pass them around the table, but I was back in the drug world, and my thinking mechanisms weren't where they are today.

I asked God to forgive me if I hurt anyone, intentionally or unintentionally, after I found out I was HIV-positive. I truly ask God to forgive me and for the strength to remember the modes of transmission and even if the opportunity presents itself, that I will have the good sense to think and not do that to anybody. That is a horrible thing to inflict on someone else's life.

We could easily change the wording of the title from <u>I Really Didn't Mean To Get HIV</u> to <u>I Really Didn't Mean To Infect</u>

Anyone Else. Isn't that heart-wrenching? Because I didn't know, I perhaps gave this disease to somebody else. That was not my intention, but it could be the case. As I learn to turn from my wicked ways — that's called repentance- I can really see a change in me. God forgives if we are truly repentant. We don't have to carry guilt or any other burden — we can take it to the Lord and leave it there.

One Day At A Time

Encouragement and support- those are two important words in my life. To deal with this disease, you have to be encouraged and process your feelings; these things are important.

I personally need support, and encouragement. For example, today (3/9/00) I had an evaluation of my mental capacity because I'm now dealing with a new disease, Hepatitis C. I need encouragement and support as I enter this new area.

Sometimes I can't help but wonder "How did I acquire this along with everything else?" It's not an obsession, but I do wonder. And because of this, maybe I can see a bit more clearly how easy it is for the concept of who to blame to become an obsession.

I believe that there comes a point in this disease where we have to let go in order to keep on living. I encourage you to try and find an avenue that will give you relief in this area. You may be waking up every morning wondering who did this to you, thinking about it all day long, going to bed thinking about it. Instead of worrying about who gave it to you, ask God to help you figure out what you're going to do about it now that you've got it. As I said before, AIDS is ACQUIRED. That means you have to do something to get it, and I wouldn't be off base to say that 95% of us who are infected were involved in dangerous behavior that led to our current medical status. It may be that someone else may not have been careful and caused us to get it, but it takes two to tango, and I know that as far as my particular infection was concerned, I was a dancer.

Hepatitis C came into my life as a direct result of me having contracted AIDS. It's important to talk about Hep C because the two are connected. It's becoming more and more relevant and known through the medical profession that many of us are dealing with this combination. Many of us are coming out of drug addictions, and that makes us especially vulnerable to this combination.

Being told about Hep C on top of recently being told I have AIDS is a lot to have on your plate. Some days, it seems like the whole combination of things that we deal with begin to pile up. We deal with so many issues. For those of us who are still employed, or going to school, or dealing with spouse and children, or still dealing with addiction, we have all that and HIV/AIDS and now Hep C or V too. It's a lot to deal with.

Support is crucial. Sometimes you can feel that you are alone, but that can be dispelled simply by making a phone call to someone in your life who is there to support you. Sometimes we might not have the energy on a given day, maybe due to side effects of medicine or being consumed with certain feelings of the day. Please, try very hard to find the energy to seek out someone to encourage you or support you when it gets like this. We didn't mean for this to happen, but we are presented with this. I hope that you will be encouraged to always recognize that there is someone somewhere in your life to help you through.

With me, having chaos in my life on a continuous basis is a daily thing. I know someone can relate; before one thing ends, another thing starts, and it seems like we can't get a breath to collect ourselves before we go on to the next challenge of this disease. Each step of this disease is a challenge. The medication is a challenge. Taking the medications on a committed basis is a challenge to me. I recently got so caught up in what I was doing that I forgot to take my night medications (Sustiva) for two days in a row. As a result, I got a spirit of fear, which made me think I wasn't feeling well when there wasn't anything really wrong. I've been so committed to taking my medications on time and not missing any dosages because I've been taught that missing medicines will give the disease a chance to mutate. Put simply, this disease is like the Pac-Man game, eating up our ability to fight off disease, which is in our T-cells. I'll talk more on T-cells in a different chapter.

There are so many things on any given day that we can jump around in our thoughts. First we're thinking about the viral load count and then the T-cell count and then the side effects of the medication (Crexivan gave me neuropathy, God help me!) and today I need encouragement and not answers and I just can't get my focus.

You feel like saying God, I never intended for this to happen. I never had forethought on the day of infection that this would happen; the medicines, bills piling up, how do I pay my rent on a fixed income, etc. I'm handling a multitude of thoughts today and it's hard.

Perhaps you need to go to the library, or for a drive in the country if you have a car. For those who can't get out, maybe you're into comic books or something that doesn't cost much. Maybe you have a support group, or someone you can call. Maybe you need to call your pastor, or your sister or brother or family member or friend.

This is a typical thing we deal with; a multitude of thoughts. When we lose our ability to focus on one thing, it's tough. We feel like we're about to lose our minds (back to that chapter). At times I think we need to reflect back to the different chapters of this book, because there are chapters here for every need.

As the thoughts infiltrate our day and come at us so fast, we now have this book that we can pull out. Maybe now I can go back to the chapter about being bound by words, or the one on despair, or hopelessness, or side effects of medicine or maybe how it was when we had to tell our family about the disease.

We can make it through. We can find a way and not wallow in our problems and be totally consumed. I encourage people to always process feelings and not suppress them. If they're suppressed, they're still there and one little thing can make us go ballistic. There are days when we are totally consumed by a multitude of thoughts and they seem so real because they are our experiences.

Even though it feels like we don't want to go on. Maybe my feet hurt, maybe that neuropathy is kicking today. See how fast the different thoughts can come? Know that I know what you're feeling, because I feel it too.

Sometimes I think of how wonderful it would be if I could have a cold beer or if I could just have a shot of scotch to calm myself down, but I know that if I reactivate my alcoholism, I'm lost. Perhaps I just need a shot of heroin to get me through the day, but I know from experience that one is too many and a thousand will never be enough.

I need to always remember that it's because of that decision to have one that caused my problem. Maybe I set out to just have one, but I got so drunk that I went out and had sex with someone that infected me with this disease. One decision — can you see where this is going? Even though you're sitting there by yourself reading a book, you're not alone.

Sometimes I have this deep fear inside me. On some days, lots of thoughts run through my head, and I feel like I'm about to lose my mind. I know you feel like that too. Sometimes it feels like you're lost and won't ever be found. You may feel you don't know the Word of God like you should, or that you haven't fully availed yourself of the services NA and AA make available. That's okay — keep reading. You're not alone.

This is becoming personal to me. It's a wonderful gift to be chosen to disseminate the words of encouragement and support. You might feel like saying "I'm at my wit's end today, but I've chosen to keep on reading because these brothers have taken time to put together words that can help me." It's definitely helping me. I can go on, no matter how much it seems things are piling up or how many thoughts are infiltrating my mind.

I'm feeling so relieved inside. This was a release for me personally, and I hope that as the excitement of these words jumps into your heart, your spirit, that they minister to you. Maybe you're up against a decision that you don't know what to do with. Give yourself a rest for a minute. Find something in this book that will help you through the moment.

Honesty and truth are sometimes very hurtful for those of us who are infected and affected with this disease, but it is necessary. Your results may have come back in two weeks, but you waited three because you were scared. Be honest with yourself that you are scared and do what's best for your health. Whatever it is you're dealing with, be it HIV/AIDS or Hep C or V or Herpes or diabetes or whatever, deal with it honestly.

It is my desire that you will know that you're not alone. For example, a person who has just found out that they're HIV-positive or that they have AIDS, and along with that, they found out that they have infected someone dear to them, that is hard. To them it's hard, so real and so painful.

For me, suicide was not an option, but I know it's in someone's thoughts right now. I know someone thought things like "I'd rather take myself out then die a slow and painful death from this virus."

Suicide is NOT an option. I did not have to do it, and you don't either. We had a choice. We had a choice to put that spike in our arm and get high, we had a choice to put that liquor bottle to our lips and lose our ability to make good sexual decisions, and now we have a choice to live every minute that God gives us. Remember, "When your rope of hope is broke, reach beyond the break."

The disease of HIV/AIDS is devastating, and it seems like it's been around long enough that some of the devastation should have faded by now, but it hasn't. Lack of information and education is deadly. Whoever is reading these words that we have been chosen to put on these pages for your encouragement and for your education, hold on. Don't give up. Remember — put this deep in your spirit — the majority of us really didn't mean to get HIV or AIDS. That's the truth.

This is to the reader who's not infected, who may think we're getting what we deserve. Yes, some of us knew of the possibilities, but the truth is, some of us didn't. We were so caught up we didn't really know we were going to get this. We didn't know we'd be chained to medicine to prolong our lives, exposed to TB, exposed to other stuff like this.

I remember when I was in elementary school that life was so uncomplicated (I'm sure someone can relate). My biggest situations were to try to make the best marks I could on a test. But perhaps, these words are speaking to someone whose biggest issue was where will my next meal be coming from? Maybe this is being read by a child, wondering "Is there gonna be any dinner when I get home from school?"

This all comes together under the heading of "When was hopelessness instilled into our spirits?" Was it when we were diagnosed? I don't think so. Our issues started long before that, I'm sure of it. We didn't have this health concern when we were making those bad decisions.

My point is, that when you're a child and you have nothing, you start to think that the drug dealer got it going on. They have cars, women, the works. That was the mark that you shot for. Hmm. How interesting. That life can begin to turn and we're not quite aware because of our lack of maturity. Then one day ten years down the road, we're told in a clinic that we're HIV positive. It all starts so simply.

As a child, even though we had to deal with certain dilemmas through no fault of our own sometimes, this was the vehicle that started us on the path, by forcing us to make decisions. Sometimes, those decisions cause us NOT to be infected with the HIV virus.

I received a phone call from a seminar I was allowed to do, presented to 800 students in two shifts. I was called with some of the responses. I want to tell you this to encourage you. All of us won't get an audience of 800 kids; some will only have that one kid in their neighborhood. However, if you get the opportunity to talk to just that one, know that you have been chosen to talk or listen, to help them turn around their life or lives so that they won't someday be sitting in a clinic being told that they are HIV positive. That's all of our responsibilities.

When we learn to sacrifice, God is pleased. He sends His angels to help us when we're able to sacrifice. It happens all across the country. There are folks all across the country who have been chosen to do what Bro. Maurice and I are doing right now; tell someone about HIV and AIDS.

If something that we say or do helps one boy or girl to avoid this disease, we've done well. We must never forget to pray, for that child in the neighborhood that you see in trouble. Try it. Maybe you won't see it in your lifetime, but there will be a turnaround.

If your plate is full of chaotic thoughts today, don't give in. Don't take a drink, don't shoot some dope or some coke, but fight. Call somebody, pick up this book, call a support group number. These are all things we can do to live well instead of die slowly.

I was reading Halle Berry's autobiography. She said it was her fifth grade teacher who made a difference in her life, at every level of school. When Halle moved up in school, this lady would wind up working at that next school, as her counselor. Maybe that lady was Halle Berry's guardian angel. You could be that guardian angel for some child in your neighborhood. It's not as tough as it seems. Just be there for someone who needs to hear what you have to say. If you have chosen to live, and to live a quality life of reaching back and helping somebody, you will be blessed.

Having A Bad Day

With this disease, sometimes you just don't feel good. That's to be expected, and you shouldn't be afraid to feel like that. Hiding how you feel just makes it worse. When you're feeling down and out, acknowledge it, deal with it but don't live there.

There are times when I have days that are just so rough I don't know what to do. I'm going to let you inside a few of them, so you can understand if you don't already, and if you can relate to this, you know what I'm talking about.

3/9/00

I need to share this. I'm having one of those moments when I realize that I have AIDS. I know it sounds crazy, but there are times when the reality of this medical condition just dominates your thoughts. I know somebody can relate to that!

I wasn't prepared for this right now, but it happens. Brothers and sisters, sometimes it's HARD. I have AIDS and it's not gonna go away unless God Almighty chooses to remove it (and He can!). I need to continue to listen to Him, to draw closer to Him. He knows the day I was infected, the day I went from HIV positive to AIDS and I know that He loves me. That's what's helping me right now, at this moment; the love of God.

With this disease, sometimes we don't know what kind of thoughts we're gonna have. I've been dealing with this a long time, but I must remember that God's time is not our time. I thank God every day that even when I fail to acknowledge Him, He is with me. At this moment right now, I DON'T WANT TO HAVE AIDS. I JUST WANT IT TO GO AWAY. I want it to go completely away, just for this day, just for this moment. Many of us have days like this, when we just don't want to be bothered with this disease.

Because I know where my help is coming from, I'm not going to go home and get in the closet, or hide under the covers. Perhaps somebody has chosen to do that. I won't say come out of there. Do what you have to do in order to get through the day, but just don't think you can stay there forever.

I'm so glad I've chosen not to hide in the closet or under the covers. I'm so glad I have brothers in my life who understand, who I can share with. Today I can make a phone call and tell them how I feel and they'll understand exactly what I'm talking about. They will know that at times like this, I don't need them to try and solve all my problems; I just need them to listen and understand. And they know that when the situation reverses, I will be there for them, to pick them up from feeling down.

There can be people like that in your life too, friends, family, whoever. They can learn to listen; after all, we have two ears and one mouth for a reason — listening is more important than talking! Sometimes we all need that. I know I do. I had to learn to tell folks that up front sometimes. "Please just listen. Don't try to solve it. You may have the answer, and it may be simple, but just for today, let me let it out."

I've had people tell me stop claiming the disease. I claim NOTHING. Reality tells me certain things, but I don't claim or hold onto them. I have learned to do things to enhance my life, and through that, God has allowed me to help others.

Today I don't want to have AIDS, and that's all right. Maybe later on in the day that'll go away, but right now, that's where I'm at. I think it's important that because we're unfolding the truth, that it be told like it is. This moment, I don't want to have AIDS. Later on, I don't know. Somebody reading this now is saying "Bro, I'm with you! I don't wanna have this either!" Guess what? It's all right, just for this moment. I ain't down, I ain't out, I just don't wanna be infected for this moment.

Did Satan drop that feeling on me? I don't know — he's such a busy rascal at times. He'll jump in at any moment. Well devil, Maurice and I are serving you notice. You have no place up in this book. You're the father of lies, and God is using us to tell the truth. We serve you and all those demons that followed you notice that you have no play in this book. God has called us to do certain things, and we're gonna do it because God said so and He is stronger than you are.

Even though I had those thoughts, they're gone now. If you're having that experience, you don't have to live under that yoke either. This is a book of truth. This is a book of my living experiences with this disease. This is me being used to tell my experiences, to teach how to live a good, quality life, even with this disease.

Even though in the madness of my early life I was working full time and overtime for the devil, and now I'm presented with this, my medical condition is not who I am in Christ Jesus. I'm God's baby boy. I'm his son, his prodigal son who stepped out there and got in trouble, but now I'm back in His arms. This really isn't about me. This is about what God is teaching me, showing me about how to reach His people and make each day just a little bit better than the day before.

It would be a waste of paper not to let folk know that you can make it, but you have to hold onto His unchanging hand. He just reached down and touched me, and He'll do it for you too. Grace, mercy — I didn't do nothing to deserve it. This disease is everywhere, but **so is God.** We're well protected.

I just want everyone to know that this is the day that the Lord has made, and it's been a good one for me so far, even with this moment I had. I've been dealing with issues that, if I had a choice, I probably wouldn't be dealing with, but I'm dealing with them. I'm hoping that as you read this, whatever issues you're dealing with, you're making it through. Take it one hour at a time, a few minutes at a time, whatever it takes to get you through this day.

5/8/00

I am having one of the roughest days of my life since I was infected. When I say that I am having a rough day, what does that entail?

Recently, I've been bombarded with all kinds of medications. As a result, a lot of issues have come up. I know I'm relating to someone who has been there or is about to go there.

I no longer have to question why. I know that God allows certain things to happen just so I can go through them and be completely compassionate towards my brothers and sisters who are also going through it.

I have mood swings, where I can't control when or where I cry, and my appetite has gone kaput. I can be hungry, my wife can put food in front of me and just like that, my appetite is gone for no good reason.

I woke up today literally shaking. I called my doctor and the advice was to come into the hospital immediately to see if they needed to reduce my dosage. I followed instructions, but by the time I got there, I felt better. I saw no need of sitting around all morning, so I left and went to work!

Side effects come and go. As difficult as it may be day to day, I know that the results outweigh the outcome if I don't take the meds. I am as obedient to my doctor as I can be for that reason. If it ever comes to a point where it feels like it's too much, I'll discuss it with my doctor and we'll go from there.

What I'm trying to say is that we have choices. To be honest (and that's the goal of this book as I said before!), I'm tired of being tired of being tired of these meds. I'm almost at the point where I want to throw up my hands and give up.

I'm not going to give up though. I'm going to stop by the job for a minute, and when I go home, I'm going to call somebody. I'm going to reach out to someone. My wife is one of my coaches — I can talk to her. We'll talk, we'll have a word of prayer, whoever I reach out to will listen to me and we'll go from there.

I thank God that I have options today. I don't have to go back to using to get through this. God has granted me abstinence from drugs and alcohol, and I've been clean for quite some time now.

There are many diseases that have infiltrated this world, and HIV/AIDS is just one of them. It's my belief that for me personally, HIV/AIDS was designed to stop me. I had to be stopped. I was on the path to destruction, and I truly believe that if this disease hadn't entered my life and forced me to change my lifestyle of drug addiction, I wouldn't be alive today. I never would have had the chance to find out for myself how good God truly is, and I would have missed my blessing if I hadn't been forced to stop.

As a result of this disease in my life, I can see clearly now, and the best is yet to come. As I continue to learn, I listen to others; not just those who are infected, but also to those who are affected. My wife is a good example. She asked me the other the day if perhaps as I go out and about to minister, she can join with me. There must be some things stirring up in her, having a husband who has this disease. She is affected. There are many who are affected in some way, some on a daily basis like my wife, some periodically.

That's another set of thought that can affect you when you're having a bad day. There have been times when I think "I really didn't mean to bring this into my family." I think about my family and I wish, I pray that my older sister wouldn't have had to go through all that she's been through with her son, all she's going through with me and perhaps all she will have to go through with other family members besides me. I know I'm not the only one in my family who's infected. It appears that I'm the only one who's vocal about it.

I know that you might be reading this at some points and go "Hmm, he's just telling us about his day." Sure, because it's important that we all understand that we're not walking alone. Maybe I'm having a day of dealing with the disease HIV/AIDS, or maybe Hepatitis C or diabetes, or neuropathy. I want to share this so that you will understand that every day will not be a Hallelujah day, but every day is a day of encouragement. I'm here, I'm speaking and that tells me I can still go on despite the feelings I may be having, or in spite of everything I have to face. All I know is that as long as I trust in the Lord, everything will be all right. When I run out of strength on my own, He will strengthen me and lift me up, send the angels to be around me. There's always an avenue — we don't have to be stuck in despair. These words should stay with you, especially that one who has lost someone, or maybe two someones to this disease, or those who are infected and just having a bad day.

2-13/01

I'm quite sure that someone can relate to this.

Today I had a 9:30 appointment with my primary care physician. I wasn't feeling all that great when I got up this morning to go to the doctor's, and lo and behold, when I left his office, I felt even worse! Can anybody relate to that? How can we regroup when faced with such awesome negativity throughout our day? Along with everything else we're carrying along with us, not just with this disease, but with life in general.

It was a HORRIBLE session with my doctor today. I don't know if it was him or me or what, but I left there and I still haven't quite shaken it yet. I'm glad this book is giving me opportunities to talk about the real things we encounter, being HIV and AIDS. This is real. This is me sharing my feelings after a visit like today. I can remember when I've been in my doctor's office and I've left there feeling so wonderful, so encouraged by him just taking the time out and saying some good things to me that day.

It just threw me totally, because sometimes I feel like our care providers lean on this thing where they seem to believe that "If you're not feeling 100% up to par, you always *have* to be depressed." I'm not depressed today! I'm not feeling all that wonderful, but I'm not depressed. Life goes on.

I know someone who's reading this book who maybe isn't infected where they've gone with the expectation "I'm going to see the doctor, I'll probably feel better." I just felt worse when I left that doctor's office today. I don't know what was going on and why everything went that way.

A part of me is angry about this. It's okay to be angry; it's what we do with that anger that counts. I didn't cuss him out or say any bad things or think about using drugs or alcohol. I just kinda absorbed the moments and as this day continues to unfold, God will give me a solution that will help me through.

I'm looking at this office visit today as a valley experience. That saying "It's in the valley we grow" applies here; I know there's something I can learn from this and that God will show me how I can grow from this experience. I've had this happen before with care providers where perhaps they bring their junk to work. They're not feeling 100% and unbeknownst to them, they're letting it overlap into their session with someone who is infected. We're coming in for some care. If you're not taking care of yourself, you can't help others. You have to have some sort of order in your own life or else you can't do it.

This is how I look at it now, though. You never know what's going on in a person's day until you talk to them. Maybe he had a bad day before I got there. Maybe I was whining today and he didn't expect that. I think I got sarcastic with him at one point as well. We have to realize that sometimes we don't realize what we're doing to contribute to somebody else's bad mood or attitude.

I do believe if I had not gone to the doctor today, I probably would be feeling better! I have to laugh at that, because sometimes we take little encounters like that so seriously and we blow them so out of proportion until it can literally make us sick, make our T-cells go down. Even with him announcing to me that my T-cells were up to 308, I couldn't pull no joy out of that because I was letting what I felt was going on with the office visit overshadow all the good things God was doing. I ask God's forgiveness for my ungrateful mood during this office visit today.

I'm gonna start my day all over. That's one solution all of us have available. We can start our day off all over with a new attitude any time we choose to. I called a brother to get some comfort and he snapped out at me! I truly need to start my day all over, and that's what I will do.

These are the real life experiences we have that might cause us to get stressed and our health is affected (T-cell count could drop) or we make a bad decision to stop going to that doctor when he or she might be the best option for you. Finding the humor in any situation can help you through the times when you start to feel discouraged.

Those are just a few examples of bad days I've had. I've had others, days when I didn't know if I could come out of the hole I'd created for myself, of being consumed by first this thought and then that thought. Being spiritually connected has been such a blessing in my life. I know how I got to where I am today. I know whose hand I hold onto when there were no other hands to hold onto. Jesus Christ lifted me when I couldn't do it for myself. I can never forget that.

Again I say to you, hang in there. Don't give up on the brink of your miracle. I know God's gonna bless me, and that's my staying power.

Somebody might be saying "I'm not there yet." Well, if you have faith the size of a mustard seed, you will get through.

"My people are destroyed for lack of knowledge: because thou hast rejected knowledge, I will also reject thee, that thou shalt be no priest to me; seeing thou hast forgotten the law of thy God, I will also forget thy children."   Hosea 4:6 (KJV)

Knowledge Is Power

I used to think that people who worked cash registers were the smartest people in the world.

I don't know why, but seeing them work those machines to me meant something I could never learn to do because it looked so complicated.

A lot of that had to do with me never feeling like I could make it. I was smart, I had a magnificent memory too, but I never felt like I was smart. It wasn't until I got saved later in life that I knew I had these attributes.

Because of that, I never really reached my potential in any school I went to. I remember being intimidated in the classroom and going around thinking that people who ran the cash register in stores were super smart folks and I wasn't smart enough to do that. I always settled for second best and got second best results.

What exactly was it about lack of knowledge that led me to where I am today? Was it not knowing the meaning of profound? Was it not knowing the meaning of succinct? Was it not knowing the meaning of so many awesome, beautiful words that I know about now? Auspices — isn't that a beautiful word? I heard that word and learned it right here in Bethel church. "Under the auspices of God...." Words have a melody to them, and not knowing the connotation of those words was one of the catalysts for my pattern of failure. That's what made me accept less then the best, and say stuff to myself like "Hey, this is where I'm at. I ain't gonna try to do no better, I don't want to do no better because I don't know what they talking about."

When you don't know something, you ask somebody who does know. Around my buddies I'd ask what's the best wine or what's the best liquor. But, when it came to stuff like trying to use new words and asking what they meant, that's when I got quiet because that kind of knowledge wasn't something my buddies had any respect for, and I wanted to keep their respect. During my college times, I remember being excited by the new words I was learning, such as succinct, and profound and all those other beautiful words, but then I couldn't use them around my friends. When I did, they would agitate and tease me, saying stuff like "Who are you, Joe College?" I knew I wanted to change, but I didn't have an opportunity or an arena to use these words on a regular basis to enhance my vocabulary. I just didn't have the strength to go up against my peers.

Education is important, but my friends and I didn't see it that way. In my young life, I felt intimidated about people who used big words. Then, when I got to college and learned some big words myself and tried to use them, my friends were intimidated by me. It was one big cycle and all of us were staying right where we were and not changing a bit. I have a few regrets, but they are slowly melting away and being replaced with the wisdom and knowledge of God.

Overall, it was lack of knowing what a word meant as it applied to a sentence, how you put a paragraph together, how these words making sense in writing, all these things that made me think I couldn't succeed in life. Feeling ignorant can be devastating. Once I began to acknowledge that feeling and allowed it to have a place in my life, I chose another way to deal with my lack of knowledge. Instead of trying to get some knowledge, I did whatever I could not to feel bad about what I was lacking.

It baffles my mind today that I was so intimidated about the cash register; even today I think that cash register people are at a certain level. It's just a cash register; it's something you can learn. It's little stories like that in my life that seem to have kept me down in the past, all of which led to that one decision that has affected the rest of my life. That's the message I'm trying to get across. I really didn't mean to get HIV, but now I have it because of the decisions I made. I want those of you reading this who also didn't mean to get HIV will ask themselves what happened, and reflect back, and use what you learn to change your life for the better.

When it came to HIV and AIDS, I only had a little bit of information. My world was very small, and the information that came into my neighborhood about the disease was very limited. My world consisted of my house and the area around it. When I left my house, I would go somewhere within the area I was born and raised in until it was time to go back to my house. When I worked, I still stayed close to home and wasn't really exposed to that many different people. There was no church connection, no baseball team or bowling league, no nothing but the same people and the same things I always knew.

My world was centered around drug use. When HIV hit the scene, that information for whatever reason didn't enter our world. We only knew it from the perspective of when somebody we knew had it and the news leaked out. It's ironic that while we were in our active addiction we were not curious about how a person got certain things. I'm sure there are many brothers and sisters like me whose worlds are small and just don't know. If that's you, I urge you to expand yourself, learn something new and get out of that small world you keep yourself in.

Because I didn't know the risk of being an intravenous drug user, I became infected with HIV. If I had chosen to remain ignorant about this disease and all that comes with it, I might not be here now. There is so much to know about living with this disease, and being afraid or ashamed to ask what a word means when it comes to medical terms and medications and stuff could literally mean your life. When you're infected with this disease, you need to ask not just what this word means, but what the word means in this sentence so that you can come away with the full knowledge about HIV and AIDS and how you can live a quality life.

Some of the words connected with this disease are so weird we have a problem even pronouncing them, let alone finding out what they mean. I'm hoping to encourage people to find out what it means in this context, so that they can pass it on to others, or apply it to their own lives. Part of this ministry is to touch those who are bound up — not free — because they do not know. The Bible tells us that we should not be ashamed of the Gospel. In life, we should also not be ashamed of not knowing. There is someone in your path that will not make fun, but will take the time to teach. Someone took the time out to teach me, and that opened up the curiosity box in my life, made me want to take it a step further and do some things on my own. I would grab a dictionary and just take a word on my own and learn it.

In the ministry of HIV and AIDS, that means to learn what Sustiva is (a medication), or Crexovan. We not only should learn the meaning of these words but also how to pronounce them so as to be an astute minister in the disease of HIV and AIDS. If we don't begin to take care of ourselves as a people, to learn about this disease of HIV and AIDS, nobody else will. It stems from educating ourselves. It's important that we educate ourselves, each other, our children, our church, our schools, the folks on the street corner, wherever we are. I recently talked with a brother in hospice care, and when I told him that one of the ways to transmit this disease was through a mother's breast milk, he didn't believe me. I don't think he believes me to this day!

What do you really believe about this disease? What are some of the fallacies that you have because of your lack of knowledge, because your mind isn't open to receive the different difficult words? You'll be bound up and kept away from learning what you need to learn about HIV and AIDS as relates to education.

Word knowledge is crucial. We cannot keep going into these seminars and classes and such and not know what the speaker is talking about. We come out just as empty as we came in. We're going to be filled up by all this information about education and prevention and we need to disseminate it by word of mouth.

Let's talk about despair. This is a word we have to know the meaning of, because if we don't, it could take us out and we'd never know what hit us. Early in my diagnosis, I felt like "What's the point? Why bother? Why not just go back to using?" It took a few years, a few knocks on the head, a few prayers from those who love me and a few prayers of my own to give me some understanding of despair. Despair is a word we can get caught up in. "This is it, I've blown it. No matter what medication, encouragement, prayers, it's not gonna change that I'm HIV-positive." That is despair. And it's not of God.

Things do change. Prayer changes things. Prayer changes outlook, prayer changes despair, prayer changes hopelessness.

You have to listen in order to learn. I heard a story once, of a boy telling his father a story. Three frogs are sitting on a log. One says he has decided to jump. The boy then asks his dad how many frogs are left. The father says two. The boy says no, there are still three frogs. The frog said he decided to jump. He never said he did it.

When dealing with HIV/AIDS, we really have to listen carefully to what's being said. Sometimes that means you have to come right out and ask someone "what do you mean?"

Prayerfully, this will overlap to your care providers. There are a lot of us who receive information from the doctors and the care providers and the case managers, and it is a lot. We must sometimes stop and ask them what they mean. It's okay to ask questions. If this is important to your health care, you should have as much information as you can get. The more involved we are in our own health care, the more empowered we become. This disease is less intimidating when you know more about it. I pray that no one will have to change providers because that person might have said "I don't have time to explain that right now" and then they never do explain it. Some folks might not even know about complimentary therapies, like massages and acupuncture and so on. It is crucial that we understand as this disease and the medications and such continue to change.

There are different aspects of this disease, and we need to be knowledgeable. While I've been working on this book with Bro. Maurice on this book, even when we're discussing things I don't have full knowledge of, it encourages me to seek out answers to some of the things I'm not quite clear on with this disease. Don't just start nodding your head okay when someone asks you if you understand if you don't. It's important that we slow down, and absorb what will possibly prolong and enrich our lives. Our goal is to live a better quality of life despite what the enemy tells us about this disease.

I was in a seminar yesterday (March 30 2000). When I came into the seminar, the presenter was talking about medications, and ironically enough, he was talking about the very medications I was on. But, as I sat and listened, I realized that I was in the wrong seminar! But I did receive just a little more information on my medication, so maybe I wasn't in the wrong seminar after all! It's important to always listen up, so that we can take it and share it with other brothers and sisters. This disease is so pervasive — we have to do all we can to educate one another about this.

How many times do we go on what somebody else has told us instead of researching for ourselves? I saw a story in the Daily Bread one day of two brothers arguing about the creation of the world. Finally, one brother said to the other "Were you there?" That brother wasn't there, but guess who was? God was there! It was a stirring moment for me, and I began to weep when I read it. That made me think on how many times I had stood my ground on an issue and I hadn't researched it for myself and I was totally WRONG.

It is my belief as I grow in this ministry of HIV/AIDS, in wisdom and knowledge and pursuing information on my own, this has been one of the most exciting times of my life. It seems like I have become so hungry for information, not just for me, but because I want to see others be equipped to fight the enemy, to say "That just isn't so; I can live. I can live even with the medication and the side effects. I can live even with folks who don't have knowledge of HIV and AIDS." It just sends out a signal that education is a key, and that I have to help educate my family, my friends and my community."

I'm a detailed person; I've recognized that since I've been sober. I know that in my active addiction of using heroin that I used to be very particular. I used to clean stovetops, clean out the refrigerator for somebody, whatever it took. I was very particular about cleaning and mixing that "nookey." You have to use that same kind of attention to detail in learning about this disease and your medications and all, or you won't make it.

And speaking of words and their impact, why did my father let my aunt nickname me Nookey when I was born? Sometimes you can be a product of your name! I was. It says in Proverbs 18:21 "Death and life are in the power of the tongue...." Well in this case,

I got nicknamed "Nookey" and wound up using the stuff as an adult! You have to be careful what you speak into people's lives.

For example, somebody might tell you "Sustiva does this and that to me." You might start looking for those same side effects in your own use of Sustiva, or maybe invent some of your own just because you heard that there are *supposed* to be side effects. We have to be careful about the information we receive and how we react to it. We can easily pass wrong information on to others.

I pray that this ministers to those who have been caught up in that kind of stuff. It is my prayer that we will collectively begin to get the right information and then take it a step further by getting it to the right people, ones who really need to receive it so that their lives can be enhanced. We may have days when we might not feel up to par, but the right information can help us through those days. When you're confused, just remember the riddle about those three frogs and make sure you listen and get the right information.

"Edjumication" as Pastor Beaman would say, is important.

HIV/AIDS And Working — What Do I Do Now?

I acquired this disease nearly ten years ago and there's so much to learn about it as I walk this walk. I'm finding out more aspects that need to be shared with those who are infected and affected. This one might seem somewhat boring, but it's necessary because it's a real situation. Someone reading this is dealing with this situation, being HIV-positive or having AIDS and working.

How does one who receives this medical news work through all the feelings and still work and take care of themselves? If you have a family too, how does this affect them? I pray that this will help you no matter what your individual circumstances.

What do I do? I've just been told I have a terminal illness. Do I quit my job, do I fold up? Do I have to tell my employer? That's a big question. During the time I was told of my HIV, I wasn't working due to my drug and alcohol addiction. That alleviated some of the problems, but not all.

I have experienced reentering the work force after being diagnosed. I was blessed in that I was in a place of recovery, which hired me to work there four months into my recovery. I have to acknowledge God's grace and mercy towards me during this time. I had all the emotional changes I was going through, but I didn't have to worry about telling my employer because they already knew.

The position I was in allowed me to work and continue to learn and make my adjustments in a loving environment. Everyone doesn't have that. If you choose to share with your employer, it is my belief that you will have to be prepared for the possibility of rejection, especially if you're in a delicate position. Say you're in food preparation for example; a lot of folks won't want you working that sort of job if you have HIV or AIDS. I believe that a person who knows is more likely to take every precaution. What about a person who doesn't know their medical status and keep on working? The virus dies a natural death if it's airborne for three or four minutes, but what if you cut yourself and the blood isn't exposed immediately? That could be a danger.

A lot of us who are living with HIV or AIDS have a fear of being exposed in the workplace. We worry about getting fired or being talked about. That's a real fear. I even had that fear with my church family. Someone from church saw me at the clinic one time, and it doesn't take a rocket scientist to figure out why I was in that section. That caused me a lot of fear.

I'm in a program entitled Take Charge. If you leave your fate up to others, you're living in constant fear. You need to take charge of that situation. Don't give power to outside forces in dealing with this disease. Don't live in fear that somebody from work might see you at the clinic and go back and tell your boss. You're a lot better off telling your employer then living stressfully like that.

There are people on our jobs who are very manipulative and would indeed use this as a weapon against you. And then there are folks who will embrace you. Take a chance; I D-double dare you. As soon as you are able to muster up the strength to tell whoever needs to know in your workplace, I'd recommend you do so. That's better than living in fear of being terminated instantly.

I challenge each of you who have not yet been able to cross that road yet to assess it. You know what's best most of the time with this disease, and when you don't, you can seek help and advice from others. Find someone to confide in. This aspect of the disease might not take you out, but it can consume you with worry. You might be living paycheck to paycheck, and to fear that you might be looking at your last paycheck is frightening.

I encourage you to take hold of your life, in whatever way is good for your situation. Some of us may choose to just quit. "They're gonna find out anyway, and I'm gonna get fired anyway." That might be true, but I dare you to go down fighting for your rights as a human being, as a child of God. It's hard enough to deal with this without empowering others to run your life. I'm not saying get a bullhorn and stand in the middle of the cafeteria and announce that you're HIV-positive, but you should tell key people who need to know. That way, you'll know that your job is secure, that you won't be fired for this and then if someone comes trying to tell on you, you've taken their power. Talk about egg on their faces!

If you're working, and you need to keep working to support yourself, you need to feel comfortable doing it. I recently returned to work for a time. This was a job after my time at the Salvation Army, and I was blessed because everyone there knew what was up.

Medication and work can be a scary situation too. Maybe you have to sneak off to the bathroom to take your medications or maybe somebody might see it and ask why you take so many pills. It can also be scary if you also have diabetes on top of HIV/AIDS and have to sneak off to the bathroom to give yourself an insulin shot, or if you're dealing with Hep C and need to sneak off and take a shot for that.

When I was still on my job, I worked my medications around my work schedule. I took my morning meds before I went to work and I was off by the time I had to take my evening meds. Now I volunteer at the Beautiful Gate Outreach Center two days a week. That's just 10 AM-2 PM, and it doesn't really mess with my medication schedule at all.

Side effects are real and can be devastating. How do you handle that in the workplace? This is why it's crucial you share with key people on your job. This way, nobody will freak out if you begin to act strangely or get really tired or get dizziness or diarrhea or whatever effects you might suffer from. Folks might wonder why you're so sick so often. Dispel the mystery of HIV/AIDS and medication side effects.

Yes it's devastating but when you muster up the strength to deal with this, please take a look at your situation in the workplace and do what's best for you. If you have to work somewhere, you need to be comfortable. Some might say "Well I'll just change jobs." That might work, but wherever you go to work, you take yourself and you take this disease. You can't get away from that; it all comes with you and there's always somebody around trying to figure out what's going on with you.

HIV/AIDS in the workplace is a situation, but it can be overcome. When I had to face up to having Hepatitis C on top of AIDS and then returning to work, I shared with those who needed to know, and I'm glad for the support I got there. I'm not naïve enough to think that every workplace is so accommodating though. This is the year 2001 and some folks still think you can get AIDS from a toilet seat.

I know there can be some rough circumstances surrounding working with HIV or AIDS. Brothers, I know that this disease has devastated some of you. Maybe your job is very strenuous and you're feeling weak more and more often. In your mind maybe you've begun to think that you no longer have the strength to do your job, or maybe you truly are weakened by this disease now. God can help you too. He can heal your mind so you won't give up.

Or maybe you're a single mom, two or three kids and you've just been told that you're HIV-positive. You've been taking care of your children by yourself for X amount of years, and now this has infiltrated all of your lives. What do you do? Do you run and get on social service? Do you give up? Well, somehow you've made it through all along; you'll make it through this too. You've already had situations in raising your children where you thought you'd never make it through. Some of you may be saying "I'm so tired of dealing with everything alone!" With God, you never are along, I believe in the power of prayer, and I pray that you will come through this situation as well. God is bigger than all our situations.

We can keep on working on these issues. We may never resolve them all the way, but we're making progress. I didn't mean to get HIV on the day I was affected, and I'll be darned if I'll give in. Somehow I'll find a way to get through. We all have strength in certain areas of our lives. Hold onto those strengths, and let God enhance them for you. We can do this.

Don't let the enemy come in and cut off our finances. You may have just received the word of your condition, but what if you quit your job and then don't have a symptom for ten years? That has happened before. Don't throw in the towel at your workplace; it may not be your time. Why quit over something that might happen? The might-happens might have you living below the level where God wants you to live. You may still be able to get that promotion, and keep on keeping on. This might be your staying power. There might be someone on your job who only you can reach, some child or adult who needs you to touch their life, who you won't reach if you quit.

In the short time I've had AIDS, I've found strengths inside me I really hadn't tapped into yet. There are strengths I display on a daily basis that I don't even have complete awareness of.

When I shared with some folks that I went back to work, they said "How wonderful! Now the enemy can't mess with you for eight hours because you're too busy to listen to him!" I never thought about that, but I do have some trying days on the job. I feel so blessed to have a job to go to, to have people at the workplace who genuinely care.

It's encouraging to know that we can still earn our keep despite this disease. And wouldn't this be a mighty statement to make: register for school! Isn't that making a statement that you won't give up? If you have an opportunity to go to school through your company, maybe to enhance your job skills or get a promotion, do it. That might be your staying power. Don't adopt an attitude of "I'm gonna die anyway." Guess what? We all gotta do that regardless!

For me, I will not terminate Livingston Lee until the Master calls for me. I will not give up to the enemy.

To everyone: I love even though I don't know you. I love you because it's not easy to deal with the different aspects of this disease.

If you fall down, remember this. If you can look up, get up. Get up, dust yourself off and get back in the race of life. Don't give up; the challenges may keep you alive. Don't give up on the brink of your miracle.

Medical Information

Over the course of having this disease, I've experienced a couple of words that I hope will encourage us all; despair and routine. Breaking routine or having our routine broken through no choice of our own as I described in my experience of my last hospital stay. When I went in the hospital, my routine was broken and I was taken out of control of that situation. As the days went on and on and on, and I began to encourage myself, and so many others around me began to encourage me. I said I began to encourage myself first because it starts with us. Our positive thinking, our reaching beyond the break and inserting a hope that we can, with the help of others, be quiet to the point where we begin to learn that the routine of life, at times we break it and at times it's broken for us.

I've recently been learning more about guardian angels. As I've begun to read, to be quiet and to meditate upon these things, I began to look back over my life and actually see and feel that there had to be something, a force greater than me, that stepped in and began to protect me from myself. If you can look back over your life and just remember one incident where you can't take the credit for the outcome, that's what I'm talking about. For me, I'm saying that my personal guardian angels showed up just in the nick of time and protected me from myself.

You see, being HIV-positive and now having AIDS is not as tragic as just hearing those words was. My routine was then broken; despair, hopelessness, wanting to give up, all these things entered my life because I realized then that the decisions that I'd made just didn't pan out the way I intended for it to happen.

I didn't mean for my liver biopsy to give me pain and nearly take my life. I didn't mean for my HIV and my AIDS status to give me pain. I spent my 54th birthday in the hospital, and I was discharged two days after that. I really didn't mean to spend my birthday in the hospital; well, I think you get the point.

My intent was never to be infected with this disease in the first place; I was just out to have a good time. Well, my "good time" has turned into something negative that has then been turned around to a joyous time, a time of learning about the inner workings about myself; medically, spiritually, and in so many other ways. You see, what I didn't mean to happen in some areas of my life (positively speaking) it's now beginning to happen.

Remember to think, think, think. Am I going to let this information take over or am I going to let this information be turned around? Am I going to learn how to take information, feel what I'm going to feel (because I'm in the natural) and then at some point in time, come to realize what has brought me this far? Who has brought me through the devastations of my life?

There were failures that I've had in my life. The tests that I've failed, although I studied very hard and when I saw the results, I didn't understand what went wrong. I didn't mean to get a D minus because I studied hard, but I got a D minus. In grade school I just gave up when that would happen, but I didn't have to.

If you're faced with something you don't understand, don't give up on it. Study harder, learn a little more, and apply yourself to the situation. Don't let the information take total charge of you. Call somebody who will know the difference between when you're calling for encouragement and when you're calling for them to help you with a solution. Draw close to someone who you can depend on. Depending on others can really get you caught up in expectations, but you have to depend on somebody sometime.

You can depend on God. You can depend on that spiritual connection that somehow time goes on, the sun will rise and you can be okay with your yesterdays and your yesterdays before your yesterdays.

As I travel out and about and visit my brothers and sisters that are in hospitals for whatever reason, many are down possibly because the side effects of the medicines they are taking are so great. We are actually taking medicines that are so toxic until the medicine, if not done correctly, can take us out. Being educated about medicine is important. Just this morning at my doctor's appointment, we were talking about the medicine to treat Hepatitis C virus, it amazed me because you have to be mentally ready to take this medication. It can get to the point that you would even contemplate suicide. I was resisting the doctor because I didn't understand.

This is my third week on Interferon and it's been quite an experience. I thank God for the ability to get through the side effects and for those who are on this and don't have any.

Hep C is an issue in my life that I never addressed until recently. Even though I knew about the Hep C, I didn't address it because it didn't seem as important. But, when I saw recent newscasts about it, I thought maybe I should reconsider. My doctor and I had discussed Hepatitis C before, but it didn't really concern me. But, like it says in Hosea 6, "my people are destroyed for lack of knowledge." I could have been destroyed by not knowing enough about Hepatitis C.

This disease affects the liver, and the liver is an important organ. I take injections on Monday, Wednesday and Friday, and sometimes the day after is when I have side effects. I usually get some flu like symptoms.

This is a combination therapy, just like you get for HIV/AIDS. I also take Retroban, three pills two times a day, and this completes the combination therapy.

The injections are quite powerful. I only take thirty milligrams, but it's so powerful. I've found out that side effects are side effects, and if you know the possibility up front, it's not so bad. I've found that drinking plenty of liquids and avoiding citrus juices helps cut the side effects. Watering down citrus juices also works — I love orange juice!

Hep C is something I'm learning to deal with one day at a time, just like with HIV and AIDS. I've been back to work two weeks now, and so far I haven't missed any time. I'm continuing to be obedient in certain areas in my life. I've made the nutritional adjustments, but I haven't yet started an exercise program. I need to do that, because it will help cut the side effects of the Interferon. One thing at a time — I don't want to overload myself.

If you and your doctor agree that it's time to treat the Hep C, go ahead and do it. Don't be afraid, it's just another step in the journey. Try not to do anything medical on your own, but make sure you get that medical opinion. Your doctor should know you well enough to know what's best in your treatment.

Sometimes we really have to be quiet and really absorb the information that our doctors and care providers are trying to give us. Being a part of our care, being a part of the treatment plan is important. I think that the doctors and the nurses and the case managers, all of those that have been chosen or have chosen to come into this field to help those of us that are infected, at some point had to be quiet and listen and learn about the different things that we have to know in order not only to take care of ourselves, but to pass on to our brothers and sisters who don't know.

Terms like T-cell count, viral load and neuropathy are difficult to understand if you're not a words person. The doctors and care providers try to explain this, but it can just go over your head.

T-cells are part of your white blood cells, which battle diseases in your body. I like to think of T-cells as soldiers that fight off infections.

Your T-cell count should be between 800-1200; if you have 200 "soldiers" or less, the enemy can then take over your territory.

Viral load is the actual tracking of the disease. Mine was over 300,000, and now it's down to 46,000. This is stuff that needs to be broken down so that anybody can get it. This is crucial in getting our people in particular to commit to the medications. One brother I knew started taking medications, it worked, and he stopped taking them. That is not healthy for any of us. We can't let ourselves be deceived like that.

Sustiva is a medication that induces dreams. The doctors warn you that the last thing you see before you take it and go to bed is crucial. If you watch a horror movie and take Sustiva, you could trip out on that. An experience like that could cause you to stop taking the medicine. We need to connect all this through the Word of God.

Neuropathy is a condition that causes degeneration of the nervous system. I acquired this condition from one of the medicines I was taking.

I take an antidepressant called Zolov. It's just a small dumb looking pill; I break them in half and that makes it even smaller. But I went a week without it once and I had uncontrollable crying episodes until I got back on it. I had to realize that this medicine was just as important as the other meds I'm on, and I couldn't ignore it.

For the longest time, I knew nothing about re-infection. People today who are HIV-positive already don't know of that danger because of lack of information. These are things that anyone infected should know about, and if you're affected and committed to helping out, you should know these things too.

We already talked about how knowledge is power. Well, when it comes to the meds we have to take for this disease and knowing how to take care of ourselves, knowledge is also life.

Women and HIV/AIDS

I can't speak from their personal point of view, but I've been exposed to many women in the course of my ministry who go through so many different aspects of this disease.

I've met so many different women who are at different stages of this disease. One area is women who are in prison and infected with this disease. For those women who are incarcerated and have this disease of HIV/AIDS, I want to encourage you to find some peace somewhere, and some contentment.

My recent experiences with these women has really opened my eyes to aspects of this disease I didn't have a clue about because I'm not living their experiences. Some of the concerns that are hurting my sisters; one is women who are incarcerated, infected and separated from their families. I don't personally know that pain, but from being around a few sisters who are or who have been in that dilemma, I felt such a sense of urgency, of pain coming from their spirits.

These women also didn't mean to get HIV. Women are generally charged with being caregivers, providers. To have this disease enter their lives, by whatever means of transmission, is devastating, perhaps more so than if you only have yourself to look after and become infected. I'm learning about some of their experiences, their disappointments, their pains and hopelessness.

I know they in particular didn't mean to get HIV because women, perhaps more than men, must become survivors.

A pastor I travel with tells this story as she ministers to women. Picture being a young lady of thirteen or fourteen and you fall head over heels in love with someone. The pressure begins: "If you love me, prove it" by "going all the way." You've held out and held out, and a feeling develops that if you don't do this, you will lose the love of your life.

Picture a heart as this story goes along.

Finally this young lady, this baby, gives in, because of her love for her young man. After the experience, perhaps they stay together for a few more months, or maybe only a few more weeks. Maybe he's conquered what he set out to conquer and he is in a "next" mode.

A piece of her heart is torn away by this experience.

This lady is now sixteen or seventeen, and once again she meets someone she enjoys being with. Again the pressure begins; "if you love me, show me." She holds out for as long as she possibly can. Again she feels like she's losing the love of her life, and again she gives in. This time, he only sticks around for a few days: mission accomplished.

Two pieces of her heart have been given to these two experiences. She thought she loved each of these men, but it didn't work out.

Now she's coming up on eighteen and has met someone else. She's falling in love for real this time (not to make fun of the previous experiences mind you; this time is just more intense than the other experiences). The same scenario applies, with the same result. This time however, a child is born. For whatever reason, the love of her life moves on, and now she has a child and another piece of her heart has been taken away. The impact of the love that she delivered to each experience dictates how much of her heart has been given away. Three pieces of her heart is gone because of these experiences.

The light bulb goes off, finally. She realizes that she does not have to prove her love by having sexual experiences. Now she's twenty or twenty-one, and truly meets the love of her life. She's learned from her previous mistakes and this time is different. She truly loves this man, and he loves her. They talk of getting engaged, and one day, he gives her a ring. They set a date to be married. As this date approaches, each of them decides that, due to the risk factors of HIV/AIDS, they should both be tested. His test comes back negative. Her test comes back positive.

I'm sure that someone reading this is living this experience right now — it's REAL. The depth of love that this man has for this woman determines whether or not he will consent to take her as his wife, regardless of her medical condition. Maybe she calls the relationship off because she doesn't want to put him through this.

Not only has the enemy come in and destroyed something that God has ordained, but now there is very little of her heart left, all because of bad decisions.

This may sound like all hope is gone. Not so, my sister, not so. There is always hope with God. The truth is, you may not feel like going on, but you can go on. You can live a good life despite your medical condition. This was designed by the devil to take you out, but you don't have to give in. It may take some time for you to sort through all of what comes with this disease. Think of it like this. Maybe your child was spared. Maybe your testimony can help some other young girl avoid following your path.

My sister, no matter how much hopelessness you're feeling, no matter how much despair, no matter how badly you want to throw in the towel, don't. You may have given in to what you thought was love, but my sister, God is love. Jesus is love. This is not preaching, this is truth. GOD IS LOVE.

He is watching over all of us, and even though it might seem like all hope is gone, God has not abandoned you. Even if you are rejected by your family, God is still there.

Sisters, nothing, not HIV and AIDS, not jail, not broken relationships can separate you from the love of God. Whatever got you into jail, there is hope. Avail yourself of the services that are out there for you, that can help you prolong your life and decrease the number of grandmothers and grandfathers raising grandchildren because their children have died of this disease. Stopping this disease starts with us. Nobody gets this disease alone. We men need to stop and think before putting ourselves at risk by our behavior and putting our entire families at risk. It starts with you loving and respecting your bodies and not giving in to sexual temptation and putting yourselves at medical risk. When I was in active addiction, my favorite line was "Leave me alone — I'm only hurting myself!" That is a lie from the pit of Hell, the biggest lie the enemy has gotten some of us to believe. We're hurting those who love us, and who is love? GOD.

Sisters who are incarcerated, sisters who have given much of their hearts to sexual experiences in the search for love over time, prop up that head, square those shoulders and get back in the race of life. It's not easy for a man to travel this road, and I know it must be a double or triple whammy for a woman to deal with HIV and AIDS. You didn't mean for this to happen. Some of you can honestly say "I was minding my own business, taking care of my family and this disease was brought into my home."

You can pull a blessing out of this, you can turn it around. No, you don't have to get a bullhorn and make announcements about your medical situation. When you're ready, get yourself some support for those moments when you're feeling so out of it. We need you. We need you to do so many things, some of which we've always taken you for granted over. This disease can turn a strong sister into a weakling. We must be honest about this disease.

Sisters, you're the ones who bring the babies into the world. You know the enemy wants to wipe you out. This disease may have started with white gay males, but you see where it has spread. Ultimately, the devil's mission is to take out as many of you as he can, and I believe that this disease is specifically designed to take you sisters out.

Find your niche with this disease that you can pull another sister through, or perhaps prevent another sister from getting infected. It's fine that God allows me to go out and about and talk about this disease to so many people, but think of the effect you could have on another sister that's going through, or even contemplating giving a piece of her heart that is not designed to last forever, until death do they part.

You have a testimony sisters — DON'T SIT ON IT. I beg of you. This disease thinks that it's having its way with you. You're too strong for this. As I heard a preacher say, "put your hands on your hips, let your backbone slip, give it some neck action and tell it "I'm not having it!" You can pull up another sister, to walk with you perhaps. There is strength in unity.

If you have been thinking about pairing up with someone who is infected because you seem to be in sync, let it grow. Continue to connect, so that the two of you can affect a third sister. Notice I have not mentioned race or color, because that is not important where this disease is concerned. Yes, African-American women are the fastest growing group in terms of rate of new infections, but all women are at risk. You can cross racial lines by reaching out, because this disease has no respect of your color or your race.

Our people do need help, and I believe in the saying "Charity begins at home." But after you sweep around your own door, you can sweep around somebody else's. And you don't have to know them to do that.

As a brother who has so much respect for you sisters, I get emotional about this. I remember watching my oldest sister go up against this disease. Even when the doctors told her "You are going to lose your son," she still fought a good fight for his life. I watched it on a daily basis, even through my active addiction. I watched the strength that you sisters have on the inside, and it touched me, even with my mind clouded. I encourage you now, take up your cross and do what you gotta do to minister to that person you need to get to so that they won't go through what you've been through.

Sisters, I love you. I know it's scary because this requires change in so many areas of our lives. I know some of you are very closed with your personal business. If you feel on the inside that you need to do something to combat this disease, do it. Maybe there's a church in your community that's involved. This is no knock on my church, but right now, there's only one other brother besides me involved in our AIDS Task Force, and he is not infected, just concerned.

If there's no ATF in your church, maybe you can start one. Sometimes that kind of ministry is aimed towards men — maybe you can start one for women. The women will be there for you even if the men aren't. Take a chance. I D-double dare you! (that used to work when I was a kid!)

If the enemy turns on the burners, turn up your pressing towards the mark of the high calling in Christ. Sisters, you display your power in so many aspects of your daily life. You deal with the pain of giving yourselves away and not getting love in return, of standing before that judge and hearing that you have to serve time. Maybe you felt like "I won't come out alive" because you're infected. Maybe you wonder who will take your children while you're locked away, or after you're gone.

You didn't mean to get this disease. You didn't mean for it to happen. I don't care what no one tries to convince you of, you didn't set out to get this and I D-double dare you to stand on that truth.

For the sister who's coming out of prison and doesn't know what to do, find a support group. There should be an AIDS awareness program in your town somewhere. Get yourself a case manager so you can access services that will enhance the quality of your life.

Calling all sisters who are infected with HIV and AIDS! Calling all sisters who are infected and affected to the challenge. Calling you to take it on, incident by incident, situation by situation. Stand up and be counted. There is so much you can do, even little by little.

"But you don't understand — you're a man!" No, I can't fully understand. I'm just being used to stand in the gap until a sister is raised up to take the baton. Some of you have chosen to share a little bit of your pain with me, and through that, I know what little bit I know. I wouldn't have had a clue otherwise.

One sister I talked to shared that she had just gotten out of prison and had spent time with her family and had a good old time. As the tears began to roll down her face, I began to truly feel some of the pain that she was feeling, knowing what she brings to the family table with this disease.

I heard another sister say "I've had enough of that — I am going to fight back! I'm gonna fight back my addiction, I'm gonna fight back this disease. It will not win. I will see my grandbabies graduate kindergarten, middle school. I'll be there to take them to the mall and to just be their grandmother."

To the sisters who may be feeling bitter because this disease came to you while you were minding your own business and taking care of your family, we're not even gonna discuss how it got in, just that it's there. The struggle won't be easy, but you can get through it. You can reach back at some point and touch another sister who was home minding her business when this disease came into her home too.

No lecture about "what good is bitterness gonna serve" here. You have to process those feelings for yourself. I just want you to know that you can come out of it, and you can be a blessing to that one person who's waiting just for you. I know that you didn't mean to get this thing — you were home doing everything right when this came to you. For you, for that woman who was infected due to rape or incest and for any sister who didn't acquire this through her own bad decisions but someone else's, hold on. Don't give up on the brink of your miracle. Read the chapter on despair if you need to. Find your strength and go on. Your family needs you.

Back to those sisters who served time in jail. Maybe you didn't mean to get locked up. Maybe you didn't know what your man was up to until the police came, maybe he didn't tell you the whole story. You didn't mean to do wrong.

Or maybe you knew there was something going on, but you couldn't stop for whatever reason. It's like me and my drug and alcohol addiction. It took me a few times of "Oops upside my head" before the light bulb came on. I knew it wasn't good for me, but I kept going back to it until I ended up paying a heavy price. Am I relating to anybody?

I pray that this chapter has opened the door of relief to some sister; maybe to one who just got the diagnosis of HIV, or maybe one who just got sentenced to jail time or one who just isn't sure of her medical status and is waiting to find out.

Sisters, in truth and honesty, know that you're beautiful. We love you and God loves you more.

One On One With Me
When I Look In The Mirror: What Do I See?

In basketball, going one-on-one is competition. Going one-on-one with yourself is different. Dealing with what's inside you is a challenge if you haven't taken time to do that before. I've been on an emotional roller coaster since that day when the doctor told me my T-cell count had dropped below two hundred, which means that by medical standards, I had moved from being HIV-positive to having AIDS. I can't even remember the exact words the doctor used when he told me, just "below two hundred." I felt like "here we go again."

Going one-on-one with yourself doesn't necessarily mean being physically alone. You could be in a crowded room and still be one-on-one with yourself. I've found myself in a room full of people and felt like that. When I'm somewhere where I'm pretty sure I'm the only one who has AIDS, my mood changes. I don't want to say it's an awful feeling, but it's a strange feeling. It's a real strange feeling; a mixture of emotions on my part.

I'll tell you this: going one-on-one with Livingston is difficult. There are times when I'm still in somewhat of a denial of having AIDS. I told my wife one day when I was at my wit's end that I didn't want to have AIDS that day. That wasn't the only time I felt that way, just one day when it was particularly bad.

When you look in the mirror, what do you see? When you're dealing with HIV and AIDS, this can become an issue at some point in the process.

I asked myself that question not long ago. When I looked in the mirror in August 2001, I saw an AIDS patient on the decline. I was really going through it, brothers and sisters. Even with all the spiritual folks around me, I was ready to give up. I had lost faith in the AIDS Task Force's encouragement, the pastor's encouragement, the doctor, the care provider, all of them because of what I saw in the mirror. Can somebody relate to this? I know you can.

Over the past year, with the biopsy that went wrong and me not taking care of myself to the point where my wife had to go behind my back and call the doctor on me last August, had I really given up? I didn't want to answer that question, but I do believe the answer is yes. And a lot of it had to do with what I saw in the mirror.

I was going through what they call "wasting." That's what people think of when they think of HIV and AIDS; someone who used to be healthy, but as a result of the disease, they're all skinny and emaciated; in other words, they look sick! My weight was way down, I was looking sick in my opinion, and when I looked at that image in the mirror, I started believing what I saw and I started to give up. I would look and then I would ask myself "Is this the day?"

When I was going through this period of sickness, I had a mirror where I could see myself when I woke up. My reflection was the first thing I saw, and most days, I started off my days depressed. I saw the reflection of this sickly man. Sometimes we're not the prettiest when we first wake up anyway. That has nothing to do with HIV and AIDS — we just looking ugly! Hair disarrayed, teeth not in — you've been asleep!

Anyway, I was really down until I was put in touch with a doctor in Philadelphia who put me on Serostim. Serostim prevents wasting, and promotes healing for the whole person, not just internally, but externally as well. You don't have to look all skinny and wasted; it hurts you psychologically to be like that. This drug costs $15,000 a year, and because of that, a lot of folks don't have access to it. Some don't even know about it. I only found out because this doctor cared enough about me to recommend that I get on it, and found a way for me to be able to receive it. I'd gotten down to as low as 139 pounds, but now thanks be to God, I'm back to weighing 185.

I've been meaning to ask other AIDS survivors about the whole mirror issue, because I know I'm not the only one who was ever bothered by it!

One infected brother I know looks like he's sick, and then there's another brother who's had it longer than I have, but he looks good physically. I wonder, when these brothers look in the mirror, what do they see? I wonder what a woman who is infected sees when she looks in the mirror, especially a woman who has always been outwardly attractive.

For all I know, those folks might choose not to even look in the mirror! Should it be an unwritten law with people who have HIV and AIDS that you don't look in the mirror anymore? That's an Arsenio Hall moment; it makes one go HMMMMMM.

I'd also like to know what a non-infected person sees when he or she looks in the mirror. Sometimes non-infected people look in the mirror and don't like what they see either. Maybe there's a common thread. It's just a life thing.

Prayer Changes Things

I have a T-shirt that says **Relax — God Is In Charge**. I thought Livingston was in charge. I thought that way for the longest time, and my lifestyle showed it. I stayed in addiction for as long as I did because I thought I was in control, that I could quit anytime I felt like it and that there was nothing to worry about, no problem.

When we walk in that particular attitude, we go wrong. We're not in charge of any of this. God is in control. Learning this is what helped me get out of addiction once and for all, and to find the true direction for my life.

One of the things that God has allowed me to become is a peer educator. That's where you're used to minister to someone who is just getting the news that they are HIV-positive or that they now have AIDS. That's a whole different area that I recently became aware of- some folks are staying out there until they've gone from HIV-positive to having AIDS. There's still hope though — even if a person stays out there until they've moved into having AIDS, we're gonna keep hope alive. If you stayed out that long and you come in and get the big one, we can pull a blessing out of the fact that you did come in at the time that you did. Through your spiritual growth and the medical community and all the things that God is manifesting in this area of HIV and AIDS. It's not wonderful to be HIV-positive, but it is wonderful during this time of my life of being HIV-positive that so much is going on.

Rev. Dr. Wilfred Jacobus Messiah from South Africa often visits Bethel to preach. His message one Sunday hit on part of what I want to talk about. He preached on effective prayer. Praying is simply talking to God, and also listening to what He has to tell you in return.

Before I even knew that prayer changes things, before I knew that someone was praying for me, before I knew that the road that I would be traveling — I definitely **needed** prayer. In my early life, I was never one who got on my knees and prayed, not as a child, not as a teenager or as a young adult.

The preacher preached on John 17 in three sections. Jesus prayed for us. Perhaps — I'll never know now — had I prayed more when I was younger, maybe some of the things that happened to me might not have happened.

Dwelling on things, and thinking on things, having a thought about things and dispelling those thoughts, like "I'm HIV-positive and I'm going to die." If you dwell on that thought, you probably will die. I'm here to encourage you not to dwell so much that way. We do have those thoughts — that's natural, we can't deny how we feel — but we can't stay there. During the course of a day, if we really think about it, we get all kinds of feelings, and if we were to act out on all of those feelings, that's all we'd have time to do; we wouldn't have time to work, we wouldn't have time to minister. Learning to pray, and doing so often, has helped me through those rough moments, those rough days when the weight of this disease and the calling that came with it seem too heavy for me to carry.

It's very important that we touch people. By God allowing me to be open and free with this aspect of my life, by being first HIV-positive and now with AIDS and how He has shown me in so many different ways that He can use me for His glory. That was also in John 17 in the sermon today, about doing things for the glory of God and not for self. I try real hard to work in this area; having AIDS and ministering to people infected with HIV and AIDS, it's very, very important that I learn how to put myself on the back burner a lot of times in order that I can come forth and let God use me for His glory so that I can help somebody through the moment, the hour, the day that's HIV-positive.

Our communities have been touched and devastated by this disease and don't recognize that this disease is present, or we look away, like when you see a crime and know the perpetrator and don't say anything. HIV and AIDS is everybody's business because it's touching everybody. Whether it's a family member or a friend or a fellow church member — if you're just a Bethel member, you know somebody who is affected: ME. Those that know about me here realize that they do know somebody, and as I go through being thin and worrying that this is it and being given an opportunity to stand before the church and tell them that the devil thought he had me but I got away once again, they understand how this disease is. I've started getting myself together again — after this latest bout with my diabetes, I'm on the comeback trail and my feet are feeling better. I'm saying this because people need to know that it does get better even if it doesn't seem like it won't get better. It does get better in most cases, and if you know the Lord in the pardoning of your sins, then you always know that you got somebody you can depend on. Being HIV-positive or having AIDS, it's crucial that you have that somebody.

I remember the first lady God allowed me to minister to that was in preparation to going home to be with the Lord. Her name was Rosemary, and she lived in a trailer park in Glasgow. Her friend brought me there and left us alone. I was a new Christian then, and the only Bible verse I kind of knew was the 27th Psalm. Watching Rosemary in preparation to be called home was awesome. There was such a peace on her face and even though she was in the state that she was in, God allowed her to send me a signal to let me know that she heard this Word from the Lord in her preparation period. As she lived, she was such an encouragement to my life. She had so much zeal to try to get the word out to people in the church that HIV is here and is affecting and infecting the people of God, the children of God. I thank God for the time Rosemary had with us, to instill in me the importance of getting the word out.

Although we didn't really mean to get HIV, we need your help. We need your love, your hugs, and your compassion. We need all of these things because we get so discouraged. It seems like somebody is always going through, or coming out if it. It keeps us on our toes. It keeps us alert that there's always more knowledge about this disease we need to educate ourselves with. Don't close your mind because one thing is working; when it stops working, then what? Let it be a constant in your life to want to have a desire to learn more and more that you can pass on to the unknowledgeable ones in a language that they will understand. Just continue to let God use you in this area because it's important. Some of our brothers and sisters are in such denial about this disease. Maybe you'll be the instrument God uses that will get them to say "Well maybe I'll try this, or maybe I'll try that, or listen."

You know, the disease of HIV and AIDS is running rampant throughout the world, and I feel in my spirit right now at this moment that God will get the glory for this devastation. People all over the world are being infected and affected. I read daily reports — even in Australia, New Zealand, Russia, China — countries are in denial about this thing. They're beginning to come out — Japan — to recognize that it is here and it has touched our society. There has been research on Thailand with their professional sex workers and how it has touched that country. I always come back to Africa, where so many are affected. It comes down to AZT being available to be given to an infected woman who is pregnant, or not having AZT to kind of give the hope that at least this child will not be infected too. These folks didn't really meant to get HIV either. Yes, it's because of our behavior and this that and the other, but the bottom line is, we didn't mean for it to happen. But, when you turn your back on God, that's when the enemy has his chance to start working on you, and this disease is one of his things. I know it is — only the devil could come up with something this mean-spirited and destructive, something that can get at those who lived crazy lifestyles as well as those who were just living peaceful lives and never saw it coming.

Easter Sunday to me used to mean getting drunk, dressing up and going to church that one time a year. I'm glad that's behind me now. I see it for what it is now: Resurrection Sunday. I've just been getting that into my spirit and realizing the awesome power of God, the gift that we were all given. I know that the angel rolled that stone away from His tomb. That was a heavy burden; if He could roll that big old stone away, He can roll our heavy burdens aside so we can enjoy our lives. Knowing that Jesus died for my sins — for our sins — is awesome. He willingly laid his life down to take on the sins of the world, and then took it back again to let us know that He kept His word to us.

My connection with the Lord Jesus Christ has been so awesome. I read the book of Judges recently, and I knew He was with me because I saw certain connections between Gideon asking the Lord to show him certain things and me asking the Lord to show me certain things. I can't even describe it in a word, but it's wonderful. I know that everybody reading this won't necessarily agree with me, but for me, I know Jesus Christ is the way. Without Him, I would be nothing and I would have probably been taken out by now, by the crazy life I was living, without ever knowing anything about His love and His mercy.

From The Faith Community: Birth Of A Ministry

" ... and who knoweth whether thou art come to the kingdom for such a time as this?" *Esther 4:14*

For Rev. Silvester and Mrs. Renee Beaman, Pastor and First Lady of Bethel AME Church in Wilmington, DE, HIV and AIDS ministry has been part of their pastoral work since the late 1980's. Their desire to show compassion to those who are infected and educate those of us who are affected has literally been an international journey, and they are still traveling the path that began on a big church sitting on a small island.

Pastor Beaman: "It started while I was pastoring in Bermuda, at St. John AME Church. I remember a day when I went to the hospital to visit the sick. There was a young man there, who was openly, flamboyantly gay. He was very sick, but he was acting out. He was rude to people, screaming and yelling, uncooperative with the nurses, disrespectful to me and to everyone. I remember my first reaction to him was "I'd like to belt that guy." Then I began to think that maybe I had some preconceived notions of him based on his openly gay mannerisms, and I knew it was unfair to start judging him."

In future hospital visits, Pastor Beaman set time aside to minister to this young man, and found that he was troubled indeed. He had AIDS, and the climate on the island was not friendly towards AIDS survivors at that time.

Pastor Beaman: "At that time in Bermuda, AIDS was looked at as the gay people's disease. They're a conservative country, and many Christians thought this was God's punishment for their sins. I decided that I would not treat him like a pariah. I decided that I would minister to him as led by God, because he's a fellow human being."

Mrs. Beaman (or Sister Renee as everyone calls her) also got a personal and life-changing look at the face of HIV and AIDS, from a different perspective. Her career led her to become involved in the medical life of the island, and she quickly discovered the extent to which HIV and AIDS had gained a foothold.

Sister Renee: "I became involved in HIV and AIDS ministry because I was looking for a job that would allow me to be in church with my husband on Sundays! That sounds strange, but that's how it happened. It began in 1988. We were just relocated nine months prior to the island of Bermuda. Wanting to continue my career even in a totally different country, I went to the hospital and I sought employment. I met the nursing staff there, and the administrators, and I thought working there would be a wonderful opportunity."

Mrs. Beaman was troubled by the fact that she would have to work on Sundays if she took a job at the hospital, the only one on the island.

Sister Renee: "I was new to the island, and with my husband being the pastor of the largest church with a lot of ministries we wanted to do, I wanted to be in church on Sunday. I wanted to be there as a First Lady, but more important, I wanted to be there for spiritual reasons. When it looked like I wouldn't be able to go to church on Sundays, I was getting very, very frustrated."

Mrs. Beaman then met the Director of Nursing, who introduced her to other directors on the hospital staff. It turned out that the director in charge of the laboratory had a position open for which she was qualified.

Sister Renee: "Looking at my resume, he noticed that I had experience drawing blood and starting IVs, which many of the local nurses did not have, and we began talking about a possible position, what they called an IV nurse. That nurse would be part of a four-member team and would be responsible for taking all the blood for all the patients. That would be every patient in the hospital (they only have the one hospital on the island) and everyone needing a blood test. I really wasn't that interested until they said it was part-time and Sundays off. Immediately I said "This is for me." I was not even thinking about what would be involved with the job, just the fact that I would have Sundays off and work part-time."

Just as Mrs. Beaman had to adjust to her new job, her patients had to adjust to her being there and being in a position of authority.

Sister Renee: "I actually was the first nurse of color to ever have this position. I had to get used to that; all the other nurses were either from the island or from England. The population of Bermuda is 95% people of color, yet my own people had to get used to me! When I was there, they would ask if one of the other nurses was there or if I was just there to assist, because they were not used to a nurse of color being there to do their blood testing."

During her orientation week, Mrs. Beaman had a life-changing experience. It seemed routine at the time, but one simple act that was part of her job description launched her into this ministry.

Sister Renee: "I was given a small black book. In there was a listing of names and dates of birth; most of it was in alphabetical order, but many of the names were added on. I was informed that this was a listing of everyone who was HIV-positive on the island. I saw names of officers of the church, people of high standing and common, ordinary people, all there together, and this was something I had to keep confidential. It was just a heavy weight to know that I had in my hand a listing of so many people who were going through. This was back in 1988-1989, and HIV/AIDS was truly a leper's disease; people were not talking about it, and people who were infected were shunned. It was very difficult to have that responsibility of knowing. I actually was in tears; I was very, very frustrated. I had no one to talk to; because of the confidentiality clause, I couldn't even share with my husband.

Because of this, I was able to really look at where I was spiritually. My main support through that time was my relationship with God. I said "God, You have put me here for a reason. This is heavy work."

As Mrs. Beaman continued doing her job, her patients warmed to her. Her friendly manner helped them to relax, and as they came to know her, many of them began to confide in her.

Sister Renee: "After awhile, it grew to the point that, when patients came in, they wanted only Nurse Beaman to take their blood. They saw a chance to relate to someone. Everyone knew my husband was a pastor, and I've always been one to care about people. Those I knew were suffering, I gave them an extra pat on the back, an extra rub. They began to request me, and I began to develop relationships. When I knew someone was going through, I would offer to pray for them or to have my husband pray with them. He became involved with a lot of my patients that way."

At this point, both of them realized that just as Queen Esther was placed in her position at just the right time to save her people from destruction, God had placed them in Bermuda for a specific purpose. Each of them was in a position where they could reach out to those who were going through, these modern day lepers who had nowhere else to turn. Both Pastor and Mrs. Beaman gained a reputation as angels of mercy to those who were infected with HIV and AIDS, and they built a ministry of caring there on the island.

For example, when Pastor Beaman ministered to the young man he met in the hospital, he knew that this man needed to know that someone cared, pure and simple. Having AIDS at that time meant being scorned by family and friends alike, and Pastor Beaman did all he could to fill the void in this man's life.

Pastor Beaman: "I just loved him, and I found myself doing something that nobody else would do. I touched him, I hugged him, and in doing so, he realized that I was not afraid to touch him. I did my final project at seminary on church ministry to the HIV and AIDS community, and because of my research, I knew I could not get AIDS by incidental contact, by touching his tears or hugging him. We became friends because I touched him, I hugged him, I showed him love and compassion.

I remember when he passed away. I had just gotten a new ring. My wife had it made for me; an onyx stone with a cross in it. The last week of his life I went to see him in the hospital and he saw that ring and admired it. His mother wasn't a member of my church at that time, but she asked me to do the funeral. During the service, I slipped my ring off and put it on his finger as he was laid out in the church. I was just motivated to do that. He was the first person I funeralized knowing that he had died of AIDS, and that began to give me somewhat of a reputation on the island; that I was sympathetic and compassionate to those who were surviving with HIV and AIDS."

Pastor Beaman had a second encounter that solidified his desire to minister to those who were surviving with this disease. He met another man, also shunned by family and friends, who was surviving with the disease and literally had nowhere to turn for help.

Pastor Beaman: "This man was flamboyant and known in the community as gay. He came to talk to me and said "I have AIDS. I am not HIV-positive; I have AIDS and I am alone."

It hurt me as a pastor because he belonged to a Pentecostal church. He said that at his church, when he would come in and sit down on a pew, people would stand up and move to another pew. He would come to the altar and pray, and folks would, on purpose, slide over. He had lost his job. The pastor of that church never condemned him, but she never embraced him either.

I was offended for him that the church could not embrace the responsibility of restoring this young man. We talked, and I told him that God loves him."

Pastor Beaman guided this man through a difficult decision. This man had been fired from his job when they learned of his illness, and to make a living, he ran a Bingo game.

Pastor Beaman: "His pastor told him it was gambling and it was a sin. He wanted to know from me about gambling. I simply told him my feelings about it, which are the same. He then explained to me why he was doing it. He didn't have a job, he had to pay rent and have groceries. When he ran the Bingo game, he got a cut. And, on top of what he was paid to run the game, he told me that people at the bingo hall would come up to him and press $10.00 in his hand, press $5.00 in his hand. Folks would win and then give him part of their winnings because they knew he needed it.

I said to myself here's this man dealing with AIDS and the social pariah piece, no job, failing health and being alone. I didn't want to give him the guilt of gambling as well. Right or wrongly, I simply said that I believe that we worship and serve a compassionate God. The church wasn't going to pay his rent or feed him; nobody was bringing him food baskets or anything. The folk at church wouldn't even shake his hand! How dare the church at this point sit in the ivory tower and condemn him because of this Bingo game he ran once a week! This is an indictment of the church.

He came to church that Sunday before the other fellow died. My congregation didn't know the whole story, so they didn't move away when he sat in the pew. He came to the altar for the altar call and people did not move away from him. When he came to the altar crying, sobbing, I hugged him and brought him close to me. That broke something in my congregation to saw me their pastor do this. I hugged this man, I kissed him on his cheek. I did that on purpose because I wanted the people to see, and because I wanted this man to be restored. He did come to worship God because we cared enough to help him.

From there, my AIDS ministry just took off. The community came to me. A lot of people came to me to ask if I would visit their loved ones in the hospital, or do the funeral for their loved ones who died."

The Beamans were next assigned to Bethel AME Church in Wilmington, DE., where unbeknownst to them, God was ready to take their HIV/AIDS ministry to a new level.

Sister Renee: "In June 1993, we were transferred to Bethel AME , not knowing what was going on with HIV status here in Wilmington. Back in 1993, Wilmington was ranked in the top ten in the nation for cases of HIV, and when I found that the 19801 zip code (which includes Bethel) had the highest number of infections for the entire state, I knew that I would have to continue the work here.

We began in September of 1994. Bishop and Mrs. Philip R. Cousin were relocated here to the First District in 1994, and Mrs. Cousin asked that every Missionary Society develop an HIV ministry. For me and five other ladies, that was not hard to do. We started the Bethel Aids Task Force with those six members in 1994 and now we have a very active 30 volunteers staffing the Beautiful Gate Outreach Center."

Pastor Beaman: "Bethel church provided us with support from Day One. HIV/AIDS education has progressed and so people were not ignorant. A great number of us in our congregation know somebody in our families or our close circles of friends who are infected with HIV and AIDS, so when I asked for volunteers, the ministry ballooned immediately. Bethel provides finances yes, but the most important thing Bethel provides is compassion, love and understanding. We have just been able to move this ministry from one level to the next."

Sister Renee: "The uniqueness of the group is the fact that we have medical persons like myself who are nurses, we have a virologist, we have mothers who have lost children, brothers who have lost sisters, sisters who have lost brothers; we're people who just care about one other. When we come to the table, everyone brings their gifts, their uniqueness to contribute to our common goal, and we're able to do ministry."

Because Pastor and Mrs. Beaman live Bethel's motto and lead "The Church That Cares," the AIDS Task Force was established and has achieved national recognition for its efforts in the fight against HIV and AIDS. However, no accolades can compare to the impact the Beamans' ministry has had on the lives of the Bethel congregation.

When Livingston Lee relocated from Baltimore to Wilmington, he had no idea that his new life would involve ministering to those who, like himself, were infected with the HIV virus. At that time, he didn't even know where he would turn for support as he adjusted to living with the disease.

When Livingston found the courage to tell his new pastor about his medical status, he was somewhat surprised at the outpouring of unconditional support he received from the pastor and the First Lady. It was through their encouragement that Bro. Livingston was able to take the step of standing before the congregation one Reach Out Sunday (the Sunday where Bethel sets the worship service aside to help those who are infected with and affected by the disease) and telling the entire church of his medical condition. Because the Beamans cared and didn't judge, Bethel was able to do likewise, and Bro. Livingston has since become one of the most outspoken people in the state, and perhaps the nation, on behalf of those who are surviving with HIV and AIDS.

The AIDS Task Force (ATF) of Bethel AME is now one of the leading HIV/AIDS ministries in the entire state of Delaware. From this ministry was created the Beautiful Gate Outreach Center, which is nationally recognized by the Balm In Gilead, a nationally organized faith-based initiative to reach out to those members of our African-American churches who are infected with HIV and AIDS.

I Want To Help, But What Can I Do?

If you've read this book and decided to not only take steps to ensure your own health, but to help in this fight, wonderful! God can and will use you, and believe me, you are needed! There are so many avenues through which you can help in the fight against HIV and AIDS; all you have to do is let God show you how you can be of use.

I've noticed that even with the education folks have received about HIV/AIDS, there is still somewhat of a self-righteous attitude in some churches surrounding this disease. "They're getting what they deserve for living that way" pretty well sums up what I'm talking about, and this attitude is WRONG. It comes from too much doctrine and not enough Jesus! Sometimes all of us Christians need to be reminded that being saved is not a selfish thing. HIV/AIDS is giving the church a wonderful opportunity to reach out to those who are coming from all different backgrounds and lifestyles into the church.

We're all God's children. I've noticed over the years I've been saved that doctrine is a tool the devil uses to keep the different churches divided and unable to present a united front in the battle against HIV/AIDS. The church has a definite role, and you can be part of it. You can visit a hospice if there's one in your city and minister to those who are there. If all you do is go where there are babies in the last stages of AIDS who just need someone to rock them, do that.

In the African-American community in particular, there is a crying need for people to take a stand against this disease, to let the devil know that we're not just going to lie down and die, but that we'll stand up and live. We will fight with every weapon God gives us to fight with, and by His grace, we will win.

Here at Bethel AME in Wilmington, DE, we have the AIDS Task Force. Quite simply, it's composed of members of our church, a few infected but mostly affected by this disease who are determined not to take this lying down. We are truly making a difference in our church and in our community. All it takes is a few dedicated and concerned individuals and you can do the same in your church or in your community. If you want to ask us how we did it, this is how to get in touch.

AIDS Task Force, Bethel African Methodist Episcopal Church, 604 N. Walnut Street, Wilmington, DE 19801, Sis. Renee Beaman-coordinator.

The Beautiful Gate Outreach Center (read Acts 3:1-10 for the origin of the name) was born from the Bethel ATF. It is currently housed at Bethel, but as God grants favor, BGOC will outgrow the walls of Bethel and find its home elsewhere in the city of Wilmington.

Beautiful Gate offers free anonymous HIV testing (via the Orasure method — no blood, no needles!), counseling, a support group. and a host of other services to help those who are infected and prevent others from ever becoming infected.

Beautiful Gate Outreach Center, 604 N. Walnut Street, Wilmington DE 19801, 302- 472-3002 (phone), 302- 302-472-3003 (fax), BeautifulGatePR@aol.com .

On a national level, the Balm In Gilead is an organization leading the fight against HIV/AIDS from within the African-American church community. Our people are being affected in great numbers, and we can't turn our backs. This is how to contact them:

The Balm In Gilead Inc, 130 West 42nd Street Suite 450, New York NY USA 10036, (212) 730-7381 (phone), (800) 225-6243 (toll free phone), (212) 730-2551 (fax), e-mail: info@balmingilead.org , web site: www.balmingilead.org .

Writing The Vision: Thoughts From The Co-Author

Before Livingston and I started this project (in June 1999), I had my preconceived notions about AIDS (I didn't know exactly what HIV was) and about those who have it. I knew that it started off in the homosexual community, mainly among white males, and that it wasn't just a threat to them any more, and I knew that you could get it by having unprotected sex with someone who was infected. That was the extent of my knowledge, and it scares me that even in my severe ignorance of the disease, I still knew more about it than most of my friends and acquaintances.

Now I know a lot more. I've spent hours and hours talking to Livingston, learning about the disease and how it has affected his life, and through him, I see the face of HIV/AIDS. It's easy to dismiss it when it's this nameless, faceless threat that surely will never touch your sheltered life, but not so when it gets personal. When you can look into the eyes of a person whose life has been altered, and even endangered, by this disease, when you can talk with them and listen to their story and see first-hand what it does to someone's life, then it gets more real.

It scares me to see the havoc HIV/AIDS is wreaking worldwide. It scares me that this disease is devastating not only African-American communities, but also the mother continent Africa. It scares me to see the Hispanic community taking heavy casualties from this, and it really scares me to see the alarming rise in new infections among women of all races. But perhaps the most alarming fact of all is that despite it all, those who are being infected the most don't seem to care. They keep on living at risk, doing dangerous things and basically playing Russian Roulette with their lives, and the lives of their loved ones by continuing risky behavior.

As Livingston has said often during our working together, this is a book of truth and honesty. That being the case, I'll share this with you, the readers of this work.

When I was younger and out of relationship with Christ by my own choice, I used to bemoan the fact that most of my male friends were sexually active (and some quite prolific in fact) while I was not. To be blunt, I wasn't happy because I wasn't "getting any." I had bought into the societal lie that tells us we shouldn't be "old-fashioned," but that we should do what makes us feel good and not feel guilty about it. Men in particular, according to this lie, are supposed to "sow their wild oats" while young and then settle down and get married. The thing is, if you adhere to this standard, men are supposed to be studs, but women are supposed to be virgins. How stupid is that concept? Unless there's like ten loose women out there taking care of all the men in the entire country, that is mathematically impossible.

In any event, I thank God for keeping me out of the danger I was trying to throw myself headlong into. Having learned what I've learned about HIV/AIDS, and knowing the extent of my foolishness and lack of self-confidence back then, I am convinced that if I had "gotten any," that "any" would have more than likely have been more than just the fleeting pleasure I was seeking. I would more than likely be writing this book from an entirely different perspective.

I figured I had a handle on everything because I was smart. I was "raised right." I knew everything I thought I should know about "safe sex," but all the knowledge in the world can't compensate for foolishness. In plain talk, I'm saying that we can be buried under a pile of free condoms and sexual education literature, but unless we have a relationship with Christ, we will not be able to stand firm in "the heat of the moment." All that book knowledge is impotent in the face of the desire to satisfy the flesh and to fit in at all costs. If you're not feeling good about yourself, and all of a sudden you're presented with a desirable woman (or a fine man for the sisters) who can soothe your tortured feelings, who gives a mouse's butt about being safe or doing the right thing? I've been there and felt like that, and I know I'm not the only one. In my case, only God prevented me from satisfying those worldly desires and thereby protected me from myself.

When I was in that mindset, I deluded myself by thinking things like "Well, I'm not gay, and I certainly won't ever mess with *that* kind of woman, so I'm safe from AIDS." News flash: there is no such thing as *that* kind of woman, brothers. Sisters, the same applies to men (but I'm sure you figured this out before we simple men did!). Normal, everyday people can be infected with HIV/AIDS if they make the wrong decisions and are exposed to the virus. There is no "look" for someone who has HIV or AIDS. It's not like the virus makes you glow in the dark or anything like that; *you can't tell just by looking at someone and don't believe anyone who says they can!* This disease is insidious, it's sneaky and it is RUTHLESS. No one is immune. You can't be too fine or too smooth or too rich to be infected. IT CAN HAPPEN TO YOU.

For those who are like me and have in the past looked down our noses at the addict (drugs, alcohol, sex or what have you), we need to stop squinting and realize that "There, but for the grace of God, go I." And with that realization, we need to do what we can to help those who are trapped in addiction and need a hand to get out.

Don't ever get so high-handed that you think that addiction can't happen to you. I was raised to believe that cigarettes, alcohol and drugs are horrible and that I should never touch them. So what did I do not long into my college life? Took a drink for the first time just to see what it was like. I didn't like the taste or the after-effects, but it scared me that I liked the feeling. I was the shy type, but with a "buzz," I was able to relax and enjoy a party more than if I was stone cold sober. Fortunately, I decided after taking that first drink that alcohol wasn't for me, and have rarely touched any since (none at all for a good ten years and very little before that). But what if I'd decided that it was worth putting up with the bad effects to be able to relax at parties? The door to addiction was wide open; only God prevented me from walking on through.

I remember the last time I went to a club, about ten years ago (five years after taking my first ever drink). I went by myself that time because I was bored. I was nervous about it, as I usually am in a social situation, so I did something unusual for me: I went to the bar and bought a beer. I hate beer! I'd tried it in college and I was NOT impressed. Yet for some unexplainable reason that night, I bought me a beer. What scares me is that it had an effect on me. Walking around that club with a beer in my hand made me feel cool and confident. I felt welcome, I felt like I finally fit in. Talking to women was easier that night for some reason, and unlike most of my times at the club, I actually had a decent time. And although I didn't know it at that time, I was walking the ragged edge of disaster once again.

What if I'd believed the lie that the devil was trying to tell me? What if I'd convinced myself that beer was the answer, that all I had to do was to keep on drinking beer when I went out and I'd be popular and I'd get a woman? Please! I just would have been drunk *and* lonely! And if I were drunk enough, I wouldn't have cared that I was lonely!

More seriously, what if I'd had more beers after that first one? Beyond the obvious danger of driving drunk, as we covered in the chapter on decisions and also in the one concerning addictions, there is a direct correlation between substance use and abuse and HIV infection rates. You get drunk or high, you make a bad sexual decision and the next thing you know, the title of this book takes on a more true meaning in your life.

If somehow you've managed to read this entire book and you still think that nothing in this book concerns you, THINK AGAIN. We can NEVER get so high and mighty as to think that our lives could never be touched by something like addiction or HIV/AIDS, and we surely can't get on our high horses when people are dying all around us. It's time to roll up our sleeves and reach out and lend a hand before it's too late.

Self-confidence. One hyphenated word, but in the context of HIV/AIDS, it holds incredible power. Self-confidence leads to self-control (another powerful word in this context). And both of these are the result of having faith. Faith is perhaps the most powerful word of all, because only by saving faith in Jesus Christ will this plague be eradicated.

Maurice M. Gray, Jr.